Glaucoma Therapy
Effective Pharmacological Approaches

To Anne and Pascal

Xavier D. Martin

Glaucoma Therapy

Effective Pharmacological Approaches

Hogrefe & Huber Publishers
Seattle · Toronto · Bern · Göttingen

Library of Congress Cataloging-in-Publication Data

is available via the Library of Congress Marc Database under the
LC Catalog Card Number 96-77158

Canadian Cataloguing in Publication Data

Martin, Xavier D., 1952—
Glaucoma therapy: effective pharmacological approaches
Includes bibliographical references and index.
ISBN 0-88937-176-8
1. Aqueous humor. I. Title.
QM511.M3 1996 612.8'44 C96-931207-5

Xavier D. Martin
Private-docent, University of Zurich, Switzerland
Ophtalmologiste FMH
64, avenue de Rumine
CH-1005 Lausanne
Switzerland

USA:	P.O. Box 2487, Kirkland, WA 98083-2487 Phone (206) 820-1500, Fax (206) 823-8324
CANADA:	12 Bruce Park Avenue, Toronto, Ontario M4P 2S3 Phone (416) 482-6339
SWITZERLAND:	Länggass-Strasse 76, CH-3000 Bern 9 Phone (031) 300-4500, Fax (031) 300-4590
GERMANY:	Rohnsweg 25, D-37085 Göttingen Phone (0551) 49609-0, Fax (0551) 49609-88

Printed in Germany
ISBN 0-88937-176-8
Hogrefe & Huber Publishers, Seattle · Toronto · Bern · Göttingen

CONTENTS

PREFACE

Since the first chemical analysis of the aqueous humor by the Swedish chemist Berzelius in 1832, literature on this topic has become immense. During this period, two schools of thought have emerged: the Zurich school, represented by Amsler, Huber, and Verrey and their textbook entitled *L'humeur aqueuse et ses fonctions* (1955); and the London school, with Duke-Elder and the 4th volume of his *System of Ophthalmology* (1968). In addition, Hans Goldmann in Bern and Morton Grant in Boston have made considerable contributions to this topic. Numerous works have been published on this aqueous humor, especially on its pharmacological aspect. This incited us to attempt a new synthesis of the results accumulated to date, expanded with some of our own work.

This volume not only reviews published works, it is also rich in as yet unpublished observations as well as hypotheses concerning the secretory mechanisms and the modes of action of a number of pharmacological agents – and so will hopefully stimulate research on this topic. It should be of considerable interest to those pursuing the treatment and causes of glaucoma.

The present book describes the current state of knowledge on aqueous humor dynamics, the foundations of glaucoma therapy, based on more than 650 pertinent references, most of the author's own previously published articles, and new data that is yet to be published. Moreover, an effort has been made to condense and analyze the available data in order to extract its essence, thus providing a strong basis from which further progress in this field can be made.

In the first chapter, the evolution of the knowledge and thought on aqueous humor dynamics is described, with special reference to the role of intraocular pressure and its variations, since these two parameters are easily measurable, reflect the regulative mechanism, and are of importance in the treatment of glaucoma.

In the second chapter, the anatomy of the ocular structures involved is described in detail and correlated with their possible functions. In particular, the external coats of the eye, i. e., sclera and cornea, the ciliary body with its two-layer epithelium responsible for the inflow, and aqueous humor outflow systems are precisely described.

In the third chapter, the physiology of aqueous humor dynamics is explored, with special reference to the possible mechanism of regulation of the secretion and excretion of the aqueous humor. The first part is devoted to the production of aqueous humor, and the three possible mechanisms, diffusion, ultrafiltration, and secretion, are presented. The main mechanism presently known is secretion, which functions through two enzymes, Na^+K^+ATPase and carboanydrase, and the messengers cyclic AMP, Ca^+, and possibly mRNA. A new hypothesis on the mechanism of aqueous humor secretion concerning the possible role of the indoleamines in this process is also presented.

The second part considers the evacuation of aqueous humor through the outflow system, which comprises two main structures: the trabecular meshwork, a complex structure which produces glycosaminoglycans, and is responsible for more than 75 % of the outflow; and the uveoscleral outflow system which is probably responsible for the remainder.

Finally, in the third part, methods for the measurement of the intraocular pressure with the currently used tonometers, and its evolution from premature babies to the elderly are presented.

The fourth chapter is devoted to the pharmacology of aqueous humor dynamics and glaucoma therapy. First, two groups of drugs are described, the carboanhydrase inhibitors and the β-blockers, both of which act on the inflow system; then, eight groups of drugs acting on the inflow, the outflow, or both systems are described.

In this chapter, the second-messenger activators such as adenylate-cyclase activators and calcium ions, serotonin inhibitors, Na^+K^+ATPase inhibitors, cholinergic agents, α- and β-adrenergic stimulators, arachidonic acid metabolites, and melatonin and its metabolites are also presented.

Among the arachidonic acid metabolites, prostaglandins and several oxygenated metabolites are of interest. Prostaglandin F2a and synthetic analogues induce a decrease in intraocular pressure by increasing the uveoscleral outflow. As to oxygenated metabolites, one of them, 12(R)-hydroxyeicosatetraenoic acid (12-R-HETE) has been reported to significantly reduce the intraocular pressure through Na^+K^+ATPase inhibition.

Melatonin and two of its metabolites, N-acetyl-N-formyl-5-methoxykynurenamine and, particularly, N-acetyl-5-methoxy kynurenamine, are potent inhibitors of prostaglandin biosynthesis. Endogenous and exogenous prostaglandins increase the uveoscleral outflow. During the night aqueous humor flow decreases by 50 %, and to maintain the pressure the outflow facility decreases. On the other hand, the author found that serotonin is catabolized to melatonin and other metabolites during the night or sleep. Therefore, by inhibiting the endogenous prostaglandins, endogenous melatonin and certain of its metabolites could be responsible for the increase of outflow during the night. Thus, the suggestion is made that serotonin is involved in the control of aqueous humor inflow, and melatonin and some of its metabolites in the control of the aqueous humor outflow.

The veritable explosion of molecular biology in recent years will certainly give an additional impetus to research on aqueous humor dynamics and glaucoma therapy, and we will use the results for the second edition!

Finally, I wish to thank Daniel Bettens, Phillip Hendrickson, and Anne Martin for their precious help during the preparation of the manuscript.

Xavier D. Martin
Lausanne, Fall 1996

CHAPTER 1
INTRODUCTION

In the past century, the literature has become rich in studies on the regulation of intraocular pressure. Ophthalmologists have rapidly come to realize that they must know how the regulatory system of aqueous humor secretion and evacuation or inflow and outflow functions in order to best treat the glaucoma patient.

Although glaucoma was known earlier, only in 1898 did the first description of diurnal variations of intraocular pressure appear in Zurich [36]. This discovery by Siedler-Hueguenin marked the beginning of the true study of glaucoma. Indeed, since changes in intraocular pressure follow a distinct cycle, an understanding of the mechanism of these variations could permit improvement of glaucoma treatment.

Soon after Siedler-Hueguenin's discovery of the diurnal variations of the intraocular pressure [36] and Maslenikow confirmation thereof [27] using the Maklakoff applanation tonometer [20], these were attributed to various causes – to variations in systemic arterial pressure [32], to the iris muscles [12], to the action of extrinsic muscles [41], to the alternation of day and night [17], to the action of the diencephalic center [9], and, according to Duke-Elder, to neurovascular mechanisms [7, 6]. The effects of the sympathetic [18, 19, 23, 28, 44] and the parasympathetic [1, 10, 11, 40] systems have since been investigated extensively with regard to their action in lowering or raising intraocular pressure. In 1957, Sugar [38] reported that infiltration of the ciliary ganglion by procaine eliminated the diurnal variation, and in 1962 Smith et al. [37] reported the same for the ciliary or the stellar ganglion with procaine as well as with systemic pharmacological blockage. That infiltration of the ciliary ganglion produces an effect on diurnal variations is possible because sympathetic, parasympathetic, and sensory fibers pass through this ganglion [42]. Yet it is more difficult to understand why the same effect accompanies the infiltration of the *stellar ganglion*, which is only a sympathetic ganglion [43].

The effect of the sensory nervous system on intraocular pressure has also been widely studied [31], as has its action on the diurnal variations [24, 25, 26]. From a pharmacological standpoint, correlations have been found between diurnal variations of intraocular pressure and the level of circulating glucocorticoids [2, 3, 7], as well as between plasma cortisol levels and glaucoma [33, 34,

35]. More recently, timolol was reported to decrease the amplitude of the diurnal variations in intraocular pressure [13, 21, 22].

The patterns of the pressure curves reported in the literature vary greatly. Thiel [39] seems to have been the first to take measurements around the clock; according to him, intraocular pressure increases between midnight and 3 a. m., decreases in the morning after getting up, and then increases slightly throughout the day. Duke-Elder [5] also described diurnal variations, the lowest intraocular pressure occurring between 7 and 8 p. m., the highest between 7 and 8 a. m. In more recent works [14, 15, 16], the lowest intraocular pressure was recorded between 2 and 6 a. m., the highest at 11 a. m. These recent observations contrast with those reported by Newell and Krill [30] in 1964, who recorded irregular diurnal variations for both flow and pressure as well as asynchronous evolution for both eyes. The normal amplitude of diurnal variations varies between 3 and 5 mmHg [7], with values reported in the literature ranging from 2 to 10 mmHg [4]. The rhythmic variations of intraocular pressure are well known; they depend on pulse rate and breathing and range between 1 and 2 mmHg [5, 29].

In 1958, Ericson [8] made an important contribution to our understanding of aqueous humor dynamics, reporting that the rate of aqueous humor flow is lower during sleep, and that the suppression of flow during sleep is much greater than the change of intraocular pressure.

References

1. Armaly MF. Studies on intraocular effects of the orbital parasympathetics. II. Effects on intraocular pressure. Arch Ophthalmol 1959; 62:145–152.
2. Boyd TAS, Hassard DTR, McLeod LE. The relation of diurnal variations of plasma corticoid levels and intraocular pressure in glaucoma. Trans Can Ophthalmol Soc 1962; 24:119–134.
3. Boyd TAS, McLeod LD. Circadian rhythm of plasma corticoid levels, intraocular pressure, and aqueous outflow facility in normal and glaucomatous eyes. Ann NY Acad Sci 1964; 117:597–613.
4. De Venecia G, Davis MD. Diurnal variation of intraocular pressure in the normal eye. Arch Ophthalmol 1963; 69:752–757.
5. Duke-Elder WS. The intra-ocular pressure. In Duke-Elder WS (ed.) System of Ophthalmology, vol. 4: The Physiology of the Eye and of Vision. London: Henry Kimpton, 1968, pp. 276–277.
6. Duke-Elder WS. The phasic variations in glaucoma. In Glaucoma. A Symposium. Oxford: Blackwell, 1955, pp. 147–159.
7. Duke-Elder WS. The phasic variations in the ocular tension in primary glaucoma. The sixth Proctor Lecture. Am J Ophthalmol 1952; 35:1–21.
8. Ericson LA. Twenty-four hourly variations in the inflow of the aqueous humor. Acta Ophthalmol 1958; 36:381–385.

9. Gloster J, Graeves DP. Effect of diencephalic stimulation upon intra-ocular pressure. Brit J Ophthalmol 1957; 41:513–532.

10. Gloster J. Influence of the facial nerve on intraocular pressure. Brit J Ophthalmol 1961; 45:259–278.

11. Greaves DP, Perkins ES. Influence of the third cranial nerve on intraocular pressure. Brit J Ophthtalmol 1953; 37:54–57.

12. Grönholm V. Untersuchungen über den Einfluß der Pupillenweite, der Accommodation und der Convergenz auf die Tension glaukomatöser und normaler Augen. Arch Augenheilk 1910; 67:136–182.

13. Hass I, Drance SM. Comparaison between pilocarpine and timolol on diurnal pressures in open angle glaucoma. Arch Ophthalmol 1980; 80:480–481.

14. Henkind P, Leitman M, Weitzman E. The diurnal curve in man: New observations. Invest Ophthalmol Vis Sci 1973; 12:705–707.

15. Horie T, Kitazawa Y. The clinical significance of diurnal pressure variation in primary open-angle glaucoma. Jpn J Ophthalmol 1979; 23:310–333.

16. Horie T. Diurnal variation of intraocular pressure in man. Acta Soc Ophthalmol Jpn 1975; 79:1044–1061.

17. Köllner H. Über den Einfluß der Pupillenweite auf den Augendruck beim Glaukom simplex. Arch Augenheilk 1921; 88:58–74.

18. Lieb WA, Gwerry D, Ellis LJ. Effects of superior cervical ganglionectomy on aqueous humor dynamics. Arch Ophthalmol 1958; 60:31–35.

19. Linner E, Prijot E. Cervical sympathetic ganglionectomy on aqueous humor dynamics. Arch Ophthalmol 1955; 54:831–833.

20. Maklakoff M. L'ophtalmotométrie. Arch Ophtalmol (Paris) 1885; 5:159–165.

21. Martin X, Rabineau PA. Modification de l'amplitude des variations nycthémérales de la pression intra-oculaire sous timolol. J Fr Ophtalmol 1988; 11:843–848.

22. Martin X, Rabineau PA. Modifications des variations nycthémérales sous timolol (Abstract). Klin Mbl Augenheilk 1988; 192:412–413.

23. Martin X. Intraokuläre Druck und autonomes Nervensystem (Abstract). Klin Mbl Augenheilk 1986; 188:525.

24. Martin X. Neurosensory control of intraocular pressure in the human eye. Neuro-ophthalmol 1987; 7:11–25.

25. Martin X. Pression intra-oculaire et ganglion trigeminal. Klin Mbl Augenheilk 1985; 184:386–389.

26. Martin X. Trigeminal control of the diurnal variations of the intraocular pressure. New Trends in Ophthalmol 1986; 1:52–62.

27. Maslenikow A. Über Tagesschwankungen des intra-okularen Druckes bei Glaukom. Berichte über die Verhandlungen der Gesellschaft der Moskauer Augenärzte. Z Augenheilk 1904; 11:564.

28. Miller SJH. Stellate ganglion block in glaucoma. Brit J Ophthalmol 1953; 37:70–76.

29. Moses RA, Arnzen RJ. Instantaneous tonometry. Arch Ophthalmol 1983; 101:249–252.

30. Newell FW, Krill AE. Diurnal tonography in normal and glaucomatous eyes. Trans Am Ophthalmol Soc 1964; 62:349–374.

31. Perkins ES. Influence of the fifth cranial nerve on the intra-ocular pressure of the rabbit eye. Brit J Ophthalmol 1957; 41:257–300.

32. Ruata V. Il tonometro di Schiötz e lo sfigmomanometro di Riva-Rocci nella determinazione della tensione oculare, in rapporto con la pressione sanguina, in soggetti normali e patologici. Arch Oftal 1911; 18:433–446.

33. Schwartz B, McCarty G, Rosner B. Increased plasma free cortisol in ocular hypertension and open angle glaucoma. Arch Ophthalmol 1987; 105:1060–1065.

34. Schwartz B, Seddon J. Increased plasma cortisol levels in ocular hypertension. Arch Ophthalmol 1981; 99:1791–1794.

35. Schwarz B, Levene RZ. Plasma cortisol differences between normal and glaucomatous patients before and after dexamethasone supression. Arch Ophthalmol 1972; 87:369–377.

36. Siedler-Hueguenin E. Die Späterfolge der Glaukombehandlung. Beitr Z Augenheilk 1898; 32:1–97.

37. Smith JL, Stempfel RS, Cambell HS, Hudnell Jr AB, Richman DW. Diurnal variation of plasma 17-hydroxycorticoids and intraocular pressure in glaucoma. Am J Ophthalmol 1962; 54:411–418.

38. Sugar HS. Physiologic mechanisms in normal and increased intraocular pressure. In Sugar HS (ed.) The Glaucomas, 2nd ed. London: Cassel & Co, 1958, p. 57.

39. Thiel R. Die physiologischen und experimentell erzeugten Schwankungen des intraokularen Druckes im gesunden und glaukomatösen Auge. Arch Augenheilk 1925; 96:331.

40. Thomas RP. Effect of third cranial nerve on intraocular pressure. Am J Ophthalmol 1964; 72:529–534.

41. Von Sallmann L, Deutsch A. Die klinische Bedeutung der Tagesdruckkurve und der Belastungsproben bei Glaukom. Albrecht v Graefe's Arch Ophthal 1930; 124:624–651.

42. Warwick R. The ciliary ganglion. In Williams PL, Warwick R (eds.) Functional Neuroanatomy of the Man. Neurology Section from Gray's Anatomy, 35th ed. Edingburgh: Churchill Livingstone, 1975, pp. 999–1000.

43. Warwick R. The sympathethic nervous system. In Williams PL, Warwick R (eds.) Functional Neuroanatomy of the Man. Neurology Section from Gray's Anatomy, 35th ed. Edingburgh: Churchill Livingstone, 1975, pp. 1073–1074.

44. Wentworth WO, Brubaker RF. Aqueous humor dynamics in a series of patients with third-neuron Horner's syndrome. Am J Ophthalmol 1981; 92:407–415.

CHAPTER 2
FUNCTIONAL ANATOMY

The different structures likely to be involved in the regulation of intraocular pressure are reviewed here according to the most pertinent works on this topic.

2.1 Sclera and Cornea

The sclera, together with the cornea, forms the outer coat of the eye. It is almost entirely collagenous, relatively avascular, and roughly spherical in shape. Except for a turnover of collagen and cells, the sclera is metabolically rather inactive. The viscoelastic properties of the sclera are of particular interest in the study of the distensibility of the eye and its relation to intraocular pressure [20]. The scleral and corneal stroma are innervated by the long ciliary nerves, and their endings at this level are probably responsible for tactile sensitivity [48]. According to Tower [42], scleral and corneal sensitivities to pressure and traction are the same, and an increase in intraocular pressure causes discharges in the long ciliary nerves. Martin and Dolivo [27] observed in the rat that the corneal stroma is innervated by clear neurons measuring between 20 and 33 μm in diameter situated in the medio-superior region of the trigeminal ganglion. These neurons are responsible for the exteroceptive discriminative sensitivity and might be involved in the regulation of the intraocular pressure [27]. The central projections of these neurons proved to be on the ventral part of the oral nucleus of the trigeminal nerve [27].

2.2 Ciliary Body

The ciliary process epithelium of the ciliary body is the site of the inflow system, that is, where the aqueous humor is produced. This epithelium has two layers: an inner, nonpigmented layer in contact with the aqueous humor in the posterior chamber; and an external, pigmented layer in contact with the ciliary process stroma. The apical surfaces of the two layers lie in apposition to one another [35, 41]. The nonpigmented ciliary epithelium represents the continuation of the retina, the pigmented ciliary epithelium that of the retinal pigmented epithelium [28]. The ciliary epithelium lies between two basement membranes –

the internal limiting membrane, the continuation of the internal limiting membrane of the retina, which has contact with the aqueous humor; and the external limiting membrane, the continuation of Bruch's membrane, which has contact with the stroma [37]. These structural similarities are understandable when one considers that the ciliary epithelium originates in neuroectoderm in a manner similar to that found in retina [28] and pineal gland [9, 46].

2.2.1 Nonpigmented Epithelium

The nonpigmented epithelium is a single layer of cylindric regular cells extending from the base of the iris (where such cells do indeed contain some pigment) to the sensory retina at the ora serrata.

The nucleus of the cell is oval and clear, with scattered chromatin. The cytoplasm is characterized by numerous mitochondria, cisternae of the rough-surfaced endoplasmic reticulum, several lysosomes and residual bodies, and a poorly developed Golgi apparatus [32]. The cells are bounded by the infoldings of the cell membrane.

2.2.2 Pigmented Epithelium

The pigmented epithelium is also a single layer of cuboid cells extending from the dilator muscle layer of the iris to the pigmented epithelium of the retina at the ora serrata. The nucleus is flat, often with indentations. The cytoplasm contains many pigment granules measuring about 0.7 μm. The granules are located mainly in the apical portion, and all are completely melanized. Smooth- and rough-surfaced endoplasmic reticulum are less abundant, as are the mitochondria, which are smaller and less abundant here than in the non-pigmented epithelium. The Golgi apparatus is comparable in both types of epithelium [19].

2.2.3 Innervation of the Ciliary Body

Both myelinated and unmyelinated nerves supply the ciliary body.

Jabonero [21] seems to have been the first to distinguish between fibers going to the capillaries of the ciliary epithelium and fibers going to the capillaries in the other parts of the ciliary body. Jabonero also pointed out the density of the innervation in the close proximity of the ciliary epithelium.

Parasympathetic fibers come from the Edinger-Westphal nucleus [47] and from neurons situated in front of this nucleus [7, 8, 27]. These fibers have synapses in the ciliary ganglion as well as in the ciliary body itself, along the inner border of the ciliary muscle, where there are parasympathetic ganglion cells as well [6]. These fibers rejoin the ciliary and iris muscles.

Other parasympathetic fibers arise from the pterygopalatine ganglion to supply the uvea, and perhaps the limbus and the conjunctiva, too [26, 29, 30].

Sympathetic fibers come from the cervical superior ganglion and from the carotid plexus. These fibers follow the internal carotid, then the first portion of the trigeminal nerve and the long ciliary nerves, before reaching the ciliary body, the iris, and the cornea. Other sympathetic fibers reach the oculomotor nerve (III), pass through the ciliary ganglion without synapses, reach the eye by way of the short ciliary nerves [26, 47], and are distributed to the blood vessels of the eyeball. These may include the fibers supplying the dilator pupillae which do not follow their usual course in the ophthalmic, nasociliary, and long ciliary nerves [47].

Sensory fibers come from the trigeminal ganglion by way of the ophthalmic nerve, the nasociliary nerve, and the sensory root of the ciliary ganglion, crossing the latter to reach the eyeball by the eight to ten short ciliary nerves. These sensory fibers supply the cornea, the iris, and the choroid.

2.3 Aqueous Humor Outflow

2.3.1 Trabecular Meshwork

The pectinate ligament of Hueck (1839) and the spaces of Fontana (1781) [38] – what we today call the trabecular meshwork – form the structure located between the anterior chamber and Schlemm's canal. Anatomically, the structures controlling aqueous humor outflow are contained in the limbus, where cornea, sclera, ciliary body, and iris meet. The trabecular meshwork can be divided into two parts: (1) the corneoscleral meshwork and (2) the uveal meshwork (Fig. 1).

(1) The Corneoscleral Meshwork

This extends from the Schwalbe's line end of Descemet's membrane to the scleral spur. Of mesenchymal origin, this main part of the trabecular meshwork is composed anteriorly of about three flattened, perforated sheets, posteriorly of about 20 sheets. According to Flocks [10], the perforations become progressively smaller in the trabecular sheets nearer Schlemm's canal, with a range of 5 µm to 50 µm in diameter [17].

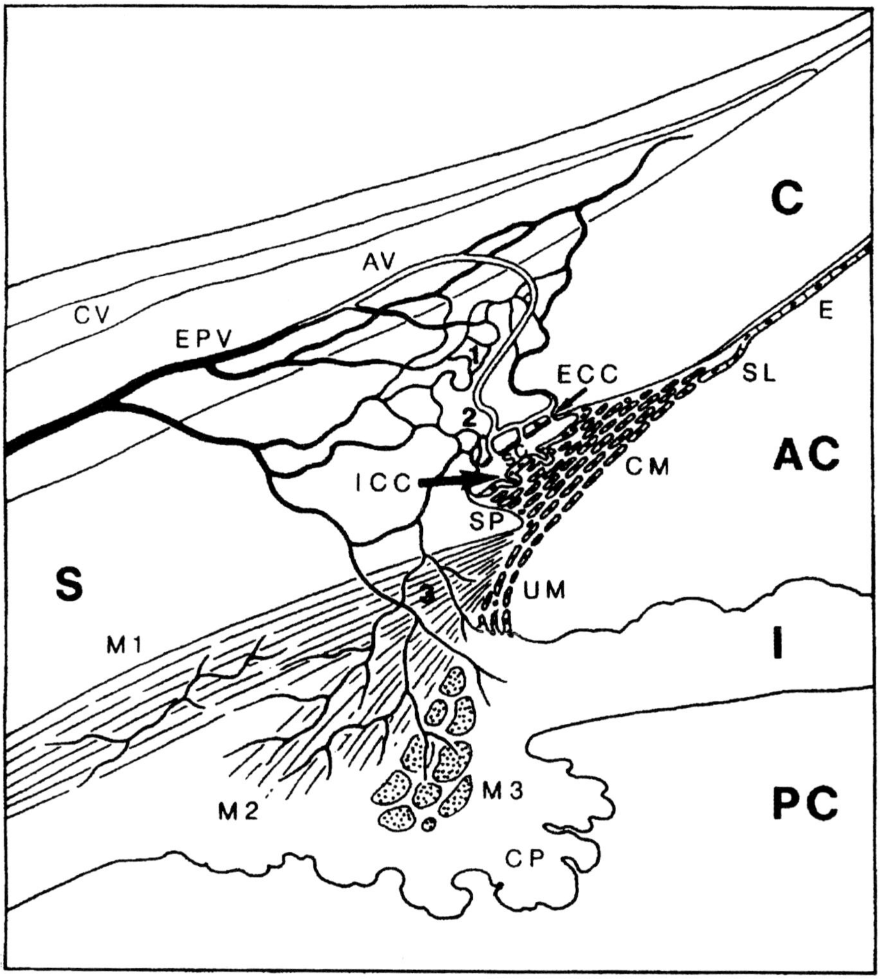

Figure 1. Aqueous and venous drainage of the limbal and ciliary regions. AC = anterior chamber; PC = posterior chamber; C = cornea; I = iris; S = sclera; CP = ciliary processes; SP = scleral spur; E = endothelium; SL = Schwalbe's line; CM = corneo-scleral meshwork; UM = uveal meshwork; SC = Schlemm's canal; ICC = interior collector channels; ECC = external collector channels; 1 = intrascleral venous plexus; 2 = deep scleral plexus; 3 = ciliary venous plexus; AV = aqueous vein; EPV = episcleral vein; CV = conjunctival vein; M1 = longitudinal fibers of ciliary muscle; M2 = oblique fibers of ciliary muscle; M3 = circular fibers of ciliary muscle (modified from Tripathi RC, Exp Eye Res 1977; 25 (Suppl):65–116).

(2) The Uveal Meshwork

This structure forms the continuation of the corneoscleral meshwork posterior to the scleral spur, extending from Schwalbe's line to the ciliary body and the iris root. In contrast to the flattened sheets of the corneoscleral meshwork, the uveal meshwork is like a string, the size of the openings varying from 25 to 75 μm [10]. Hereafter, aqueous humor can enter the extracellular spaces of the ciliary body and pass into the suprachoroidal space and finally in the vortex system of the veins and possibly through the sclera, as well [44].

Innervation of the Trabecular Meshwork

According to Ruskell [31], one can observe two kinds of nerves in the trabecular meshwork: the transit nerves going to the cornea and the nerves with nerve endings in the trabecular meshwork. The sympathetic nerves originate from the superior sympathetic ganglion, the parasympathetic from the ciliary ganglion (and perhaps from the pterygopalatine ganglion and the ganglion cells of the ciliary body), and, finally, the sensory nerves from the trigeminal ganglion.

2.3.2 Schlemm's Canal

Embryologically, Schlemm's canal derives from endothelium cells similar to corneal endothelium and from extensions of the collector-channel plexus [34]. Schlemm's canal is a circular channel lying in the outer portion of the internal scleral sulcus. Its wall is comprised of endothelial cells surrounded by connective tissue, like a vein. The length of the channel is about 36–40 mm, its mean diameter 0.4 mm [1, 18].

Schlemm's canal possesses an internal collector channel and is connected to episceral and conjunctival veins through the external collector channels, the intrascleral venous plexus, the deep scleral plexus, and the aqueous veins.

2.3.3 Canalicular System

(1) Internal Collector Channels

These were first described by Sondermann in 1933 [36] and since then by many other authors [4, 11, 39, 40, 45]. Today we know, according to Hogan et al. [17], that there is no direct connection between the internal collector channels and the anterior chamber. Therefore, these channels are probably diverticulae of Schlemm's canal which serve to increase the total surface area of the inner wall.

(2) External Collector Channels

These channels, 20 to 35 in number, connect Schlemm's canal to the episcleral veins either through the deep scleral plexus or through the aqueous veins.

They form the main drainage for the aqueous humor flow. The structure is the same as that of Schlemm's canal.

(3) Intrascleral Venous Plexus and Deep Scleral Plexus

Aqueous humor and venous blood mix in these plexuses, which connect Schlemm's canal, the anterior ciliary vein, and the episcleral veins [5, 16, 24].

(4) Aqueous Veins

Though Leber (1903) [24], Graves (1934) [14, 15], and Lowenstein (1940) [25] initially observed these veins, Ascher (1942) [2, 3] and Goldmann (1946) [12, 13] are attributed the first extensive descriptions of the aqueous veins. The number of aqueous veins seems variable: Between two and six are normally visible in the living eye, though according to Kleinert [22, 23], after injection of fluorescein into the anterior chamber under pressure, from 5 to 14 aqueous veins can be observed. These veins are located in the infero-nasal quadrant, the largest, however, being located on the horizontal meridian. After injection of fluorescein into the anterior chamber, other veins as well as some anastomoses become visible around the total circumference.

From a histological point of view, the structure of the aqueous veins is similar to that of Schlemm's canal, viz., identical to the veins carrying blood [33].

(5) Episcleral and Conjunctival Veins

According to Tripathi [43], most of the aqueous vessels rejoin the episcleral veins and, finally, the anterior ciliary veins. A few cross the subconjunctival tissue and join the conjunctival veins.

References

1. Amsler M, Verrey F, Huber A. Le dispositif de drainage de l'homme. In Amsler M, Verrey F, Huber A (eds.) L'Humeur aqueuse et ses fonctions. Paris: Masson, 1955; 43.
2. Asher KW. Aqueous veins. Am J Ophthalmol 1942; 25:31–38.
3. Asher KW. Glaucoma and aqueous veins. Am J Ophthalmol 1942; 25:1301–1315.
4. Ashton N, Brini A, Smith R. Anatomical studies of trabecular meshwork of normal human eye. Brit J Ophthalmol 1956; 40:257–282.
5. Ashton N. Anatomical study of Schlemm's canal and aqueous veins by means of Neoprene casts. Part I. Aqueous veins. Brit J Ophthalmol 1951; 35:291–303.
6. Bryson JM, Wolter JR, O'Keefe NTh. Ganglion cells in the human ciliary body. Arch Ophthalmol 1966; 75:57–60.
7. Burde RM, Williams F. Parasympathetic nuclei. Brain Res 1989; 498:371–375.

8. Burde RM. Direct parasympathetic pathway to the eye: revisited. Brain Res 1988; 463:158–162.

9. Flight WFG. Morphological and functional comparison between the retina and the pineal organ of lower vertebrates. In Kappers JA, Pévet P (eds.) The pineal gland of vertebrates including man (Progress in Brain Research, Vol. 52). Amsterdam: Elsevier, North-Holland Biomedical Press, 1979; pp. 131–139.

10. Flocks M. The anatomy of the trabecular meshwork as seen in tangential section. Arch Ophthalmol 1956; 56:708–718.

11. François J, Neetens A, Collette JM. Microradiographic study of the inner wall of Schlemm's canal. Am J Ophthalmol 1955; 40:491–500.

12. Goldmann H. Abfluß des Kammerwassers beim Menschen. Ophthalmologica 1946; 111:146–152.

13. Goldmann H. Weitere Mitteilung über den Abfluß des Kammerwassers beim Menschen. Ophthalmologica 1946; 112:343–349.

14. Graves B. Certain clinical features of the normal limbus. I. Brit J Ophthalmol 1934; 18:305–341.

15. Graves B. Certain clinical features of the normal limbus. II. Brit J Ophthalmol 1934; 18:369–387.

16. Henderson T. The venous connections of Schlemm's canal. Trans Ophthalmol Soc Unit King 1908; 28:167–175.

17. Hogan MH, Alvarado JA, Weddell JE. The limbus. In Hogan MH, Alvarado JA, Weddell JE (eds.) Histology of the human eye. Philadelphia: WB Saunders, 1971, pp. 145–155.

18. Hogan MH, Alvarado JA, Weddell JE. The limbus. In Hogan MH, Alvarado JA, Weddell JE (eds.) Histology of the human eye. Philadelphia: WB Saunders, 1971, p. 138.

19. Hogan MH, Alvarado JA, Weddell JE. Ciliary body and posterior chamber. In Hogan MH, Alvarado JA, Weddell JE (eds.) Histology of the human eye. Philadelphia: WB Saunders, 1971, p. 297.

20. Hogan MH, Alvarado JA, Weddell JE. The sclera. In Hogan MH, Alvarado JA, Weddell JE (eds.) Histology of the human eye. Philadelphia: WB Saunders, 1971, pp. 183–201.

21. Jabonero V. L'écoulement de l'humeur aqueuse. In Amsler M, Verrey F, Huber A (eds.) L'humeur aqueuse et ses fonctions. Paris: Masson, 1955, pp. 64–65.

22. Kleinert H. Der Abfluß des Kammerwassers in den epibulbären Venen. II. Die pulsierenden Kammerwassergefäße. Albrecht v Graefe's Arch Ophthalmol 1952; 152:587–608.

23. Kleinert H. Der sichtbare Abfluß des Kammerwassers in den epibulbären Venen. I. Albrecht v Graefe's Arch Ophthalmol 1951; 152:278–299.

24. Leber Th. Das Ciliar- oder Aderhautgefäßsystem. In Saemisch T (ed.) Graefe-Saemisch, Handbuch der gesamten Augenheilkunde, Vol. II/2, Chap. 11. Leipzig: Verlag von Wilhelm Engelmann, 1903, pp. 33–78.

25. Lowenstein A. Lipoid (?) droplets in the episclera as a regular change with age. Ophthalmologica 1940; 100:345–350.

26. Martin X, Dolivo M. Marquage des neurones pré- et post-ganglionnaires sensitifs, sympathiques et parasympathiques de l'oeil du rat à l'aide de l'herpesvirus suis. Klin Mbl Augenheilk 1983; 182:512–513.

27. Martin X, Dolivo M. Neuronal and transneuronal tracing in the trigeminal system of the rat using the herpes virus suis. Brain Res 1983; 273:253–276.

28. Ozanics V, Jakobiec FA. Prenatal development of the eye and its adnexa. In Duane TD, Jaeger EA (eds.) Biomedical foundations of ophthalmology, Vol. 1, Chap. 13. Philadelphia: Harper and Row, 1982, pp. 1–35.

29. Ruskell GL. An ocular parasympathetic nerve pathway of facial nerve origin and its influence on intraocular pressure. Exp Eye Res 1970; 10:319–330.

30. Ruskell GL. Facial parasympathetic innervation of the choroidal blood-vessels in monkeys. Exp Eye Res 1971; 12:166–172.

31. Ruskell GL. The source of nerve fibres of the trabeculae and adjacent structures in monkey eyes. Exp Eye Res 1976; 23:449–459.

32. Saraux H, Lemasson Ch, Offret H, Renard G. Corps ciliaire. In Saraux H, Lemasson Ch, Offret H, Renard G (eds.) Anatomie et histologie de l'oeil. Paris: Masson, 1982, p. 153.

33. Saraux H, Lemasson Ch, Offret H, Renard G. Région de l'angle irido-cornéen. In Saraux H, Lemasson Ch, Offret H, Renard G (eds.) Anatomie et histologie de l'oeil. Paris: Masson, 1982, p. 163.

34. Smelser GK, Ozanics V. The development of the trabecular meshwork in primate eyes. Am J Ophthalmol 1971; 71:366–385.

35. Smelser GK. Electron microscopy of typical epithelial cell and of the normal human ciliary process. Trans Am Acad Ophthalmol Otol 1966; 70:738–754

36. Sondermann R. Über Entstehung, Morphologie und Funktion des Schlemmschen Kanals. Acta Ophthalmol 1933; 11:280–301.

37. Streeten BW. Ciliary body. In Duane TD, Jaeger EA (eds.) Biomedical foundations of ophthalmology, vol. 1, Chap. 2. Philadelphia: Harper and Row, 1982, pp. 4–14.

38. Testut L. Sens de la vue (oeil et ses annexes). In Testut L (ed.) Traité d'anatomie humaine, 5th ed, Vol. 3. Paris: Octave Doin, 1905, pp. 434–436.

39. Theobald GD. Schlemm's canal its anastomosis and anatomic relations. Trans Am Ophthalmol Soc 1934; 32:574–595.

40. Thomassen TL, Bakken K. Anatomical investigations into the exit canals of aqueous humour. A preliminary report. Acta Ophthalmol 1951; 29:257–268.

41. Tormey JMcD. The ciliary epithelium: An attempt to correlate structure and function. Trans Am Acad Ophthalmol Otol 1966; 70:755–766.

42. Tower SS. Unit for sensory reception in the cornea. J Neurophysiol 1940; 3:486–500.

43. Tripathi RC. The functional morphology of the outflow systems of ocular and cerebrospinal fluids. Exp Eye Res 1977; 5(Suppl):65–116.

44. Tripathi RC, Tripathi B. Functional anatomy of the anterior chamber angle. In Tasman W, Jaeger EA (eds.) Duane's biomedical foundations of ophthalmology, Vol. 1, Chap. 10. Philadelphia: J.B. Lippincott Company, 1980, p. 81.

45. Unger HH, Rohen JW. Studies on the histology of the inner wall of the Schlemm's canal. Am J Ophthalmol 1959; 48: 204–210.

46. Wiechmann AF. Melatonin: Parallels in pineal gland and retina. Exp Eye Res 1986; 42:507–527.

47. Williams PL, Warwick R. The oculomotor nerve. In Williams PL, Warwick R (eds.) Functional neuroanatomy of man. Edinburgh: Churchill Livingstone, 1975, pp. 999–1000.

48. Zander E, Weddell G. Observations on the innervation of the cornea. J Anat (London) 1951; 85:68–99.

CHAPTER 3
THE PHYSIOLOGY OF AQUEOUS HUMOR DYNAMICS

Aqueous humor is a watery solution that is circulated continuously from the posterior chamber of the eye to the anterior chamber and evacuated throughout the trabecular meshwork, the inner wall of Schlemm's canal, Schlemm's canal itself, and the canalicular system, as well as throughout the uveoscleral structures. This fluid has several indispensable functions:

1. *Nutrition*: Aqueous humor transmits the nutrients and oxygen for the avascular structures such as the posterior cornea, the crystalline lens, and the vitreous and possibly other structures of the eye. Furthermore, it permits the evacuation of waste into the venous and lymphatic systems.
2. *Transport*: Aqueous humor transports the neurotransmitters mainly in the anterior part of the eye.
3. *Ophthalmotonus*: Under physiological conditions, aqueous humor maintains the intraocular volume and pressure in a range permitting the normal function of the eye.
4. *Optical features*: Normal nutrition, transport mechanisms, and ophthalmotonus are responsible for the conservation of the shape and transparency of the optical media.
5. *Pathological conditions*: Aqueous humor permits inflammatory cells and mediators to circulate in the eye as well as drugs to be distributed in different structures.

3.1 Production of Aqueous Humor (Inflow System)

Aqueous humor is formed by the ciliary processes. It seems to be derived from the plasma and formed by means of three possible mechanisms: diffusion, ultrafiltration, and secretion or active transport. While the first two mechanisms are arguable, the third has been proved (see below, 3.1.3 Secretion).

3.1.1 Diffusion

Diffusion of lipid-soluble substances transported through the lipid parts of the tissues between the capillaries and the posterior chamber would appear to be theoretically possible. However, a concentration gradient across the membrane is necessary, and the maintenance thereof requires energy. Therefore, if diffusion participates in aqueous humor production, it depends on an active mechanism of energy contribution.

3.1.2 Ultrafiltration

Although Duke-Elder [53] claimed that, based on simple hydrodynamic and osmotic factors, particularly those of the ciliary processes with their high hydrostatic pressure, there was indisputable evidence that a process of ultrafiltration from the capillaries is involved in the formation of the aqueous humor, today this appears incorrect. Indeed, several experimental investigations indicate that ultrafiltration does not participate at all in aqueous humor formation.

Bill [29, 32], followed by Cole [43], measured values from 25 to 33 mmHg for the capillary hydrostatic pressure in the ciliary processes. However, according to Green et al. [80], the capillary pressure necessary to induce ultrafiltration is 50 mmHg. Thus, ultrafiltration does not seem to be a possible mechanism for aqueous humor formation in rabbit and monkeys.

According to Cole [43], ouabain, dinitrophenol, and fluoroacetate each reduce the rate of aqueous formation inhibition of Na^+K^+-ATPase activity in the nonpigmented cells of the ciliary epithelium. Acetazolamide also could exert an indirect inhibition of the Na^+K^+-ATPase activity through a change in the intracellular pH. Cole therefore concluded that some 70–80% of aqueous humor formation is due to active transport.

More recently, Brodwall and Fischbarg [36] observed that the hydraulic conductivity of rabbit ciliary epithelium is very low – 18 times lower in fact than that measured by Green and Pederson [80]. They concluded that the notion of aqueous humor production by means of ultrafiltration could not be supported in this animal.

3.1.3 Secretion

According to Adler [1], Friedenwald and coworkers elucidated the secretory process in the ciliary body [64]. Friedenwald thought the potential difference of oxydo-reduction between the stroma and the epithelium of the ciliary body was the source of the necessary energy for the transport of cations and water from the stroma to the epithelium, and for the transport of the anions from the epithelium to the stoma. This mechanism results in an increase of concentration of $NaHCO_3$, inducing the hypertonicity of the aqueous humor and, secondarily, in an osmotic water flow.

Amsler [4] and Heinzen [89], however, observed that the acetazolamide that inhibited the carbonic anhydrase did not significantly decrease the concentration of Na^+ in aqueous humor, so that Amsler suggested that the bicarbonate could not be the main electrolyte involved in the secretion mechanism of aqueous humor. Later, Davson et al. [48, 49] confirmed this point using a comparable method.

Today, we know that the membrane potential is not the *cause* but rather the *consequence* of the active transports of ions across the cell membrane, and that an electrogenic pump [55], the sodium-potassium pump, exists. The pump responsible for the coupled active transport of Na^+ out of the cells and K^+ into the cells is a unique protein in the cell membrane: an adenosine triphosphatase, that is to say, an enzyme that catalyzes the hydrolysis of ATP to adenosine diphosphate (ADP) and that is activated by Na^+ and K^+. Consequently, it has become known as sodium-potassium-activated adenosine triphosphatase (Na^+K^+-ATPase) [66]. The hydrolysis of adenosine triphosphate (ATP) by Na^+K^+-ATPase provides energy to the sodium-potassium pump. According to Thomas [167], one out of every three sodium ions is transported electrogenically, the other two being presumably exchanged for potassium ions.

(1) Na^+K^+-ATPase

Na^+K^+-ATPase has been localized in nonpigmented ciliary epithelium of the rabbit, cat, and human eyes with both histochemical [42, 150] and electron-microscopical [107] methods. Shiose et al. [161] observed a more precise localization. They reported that Na^+K^+-ATPase was found predominantly in the basolateral infoldings of the nonpigmented epithelial cells of the rabbit ciliary processes, but also in basal infoldings of the pigmented epithelium. On the other hand, Becker [20] reported that pretreatment of ciliary epithelium with ouabain or vanadate reduced the accumulation of reaction products.

Na^+K^+-ATPase can be inhibited by many different products like cardiac glycosides, dinitrophenol [44], vanadate [20], and possibly acetazolamide through pH changes and β-blockers through indoleamines antagonism (see section 4.2.2.1). Therefore, this enzyme is of particular interest in pharmacological studies of aqueous humor dynamics.

If the inactivation of Na^+K^+-ATPase is of pharmacological interest, its activation is of importance physiologically. Indeed, Coffee et al. [41] reported in 1971 that norepinephrine stimulated ATPase activity in lymphocyte and neutrophilic membranes. Two years later, Yoshimura [195] showed that

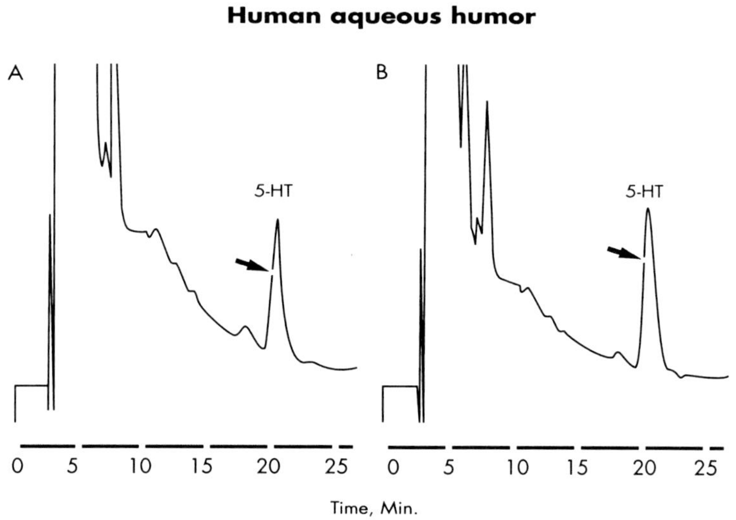

Figure 2. Human aqueous humor.
A. Chromatogram of a sample with 0.005 M $HClO_4$ (50% aqueous humor/ 50% 0.005 M HClO4).
The open section in the serotonin peak indicates the 20-minute elution time printed by the recorder (arrow); 5-HT = 5-hydroxytrypatamine = serotonin.
B. Chromatogram of sample-plus-serotonin standard 14.3 ng/ml).
Overlapping between sample and serotonin standard peaks is perfect. Moreover, the elution times, as indicated by the arrows, are identical.

Na^+K^+-ATPase in rat brain could be activated by norepinephrine, dopamine, and serotonin.

Norepinephrine, dopamine, and serotonin are present in aqueous humor. However, the serotonin concentration [125] is about 50 ng/ml in human aqueous humor (Fig. 2) versus 1 ng/ml for the norepinephrine [44, 163], that is, 50 times less and 0.2 ng/ml for dopamine [57], that is, 250 times less. Since indoleamines produced by the ciliary body (Fig. 3) seem to have a circadian rhythm in aqueous humor in humans [124], serotonin occurs in high concentrations in the morning and melatonin in very small concentrations; it is possible that serotonin secreted by the ciliary epithelium induces an activation of the Na^+K^+-ATPase and, thus, the morning increase of the aqueous humor production measured by Ericson [56].

Although Luly et al. [126] reported that epinephrine reduced Na^+K^+-ATPase activity, today it seems more likely that its main effect is to activate this enzyme [39].

In a study of the comparative effects of epinephrine, timolol, and acetazolamide on aqueous flow during the 24-hour cycle, Topper and Brubaker [168]

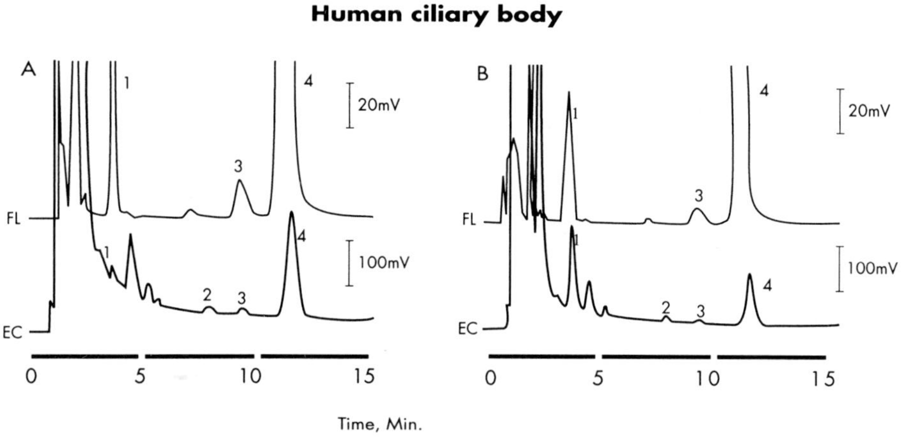

Figure 3. Human ciliary body.
A. Chromatogram of ciliary body extract
Half of the ciliary body from a freshly enucleated human eye was homogenized in 200 ml HPLC pure water and centrifuged for 2.5 minutes at 3,500 rpm. Then, 25 ml of supernatant were injected into an HPLC-system coupled with simultaneous fluorescence (FL) and electrochemical detection (EC). The 5-L-hydroxytryptophan (1) concentration was between 3.6 and 4.3 ng/ml in the supernatant. L-tryptophan (4), serotonin (3), and 5-hydroxyindolacetic acid (2) were also detected.
B. Chromatogram of the ciliary body extract (50%) plus 5-L-hydroxytryptophan standard (50%)
That is to say, 50% supernatant ciliary body and 50% standard containing 625 pg of 5-L-hydroxytryptophan.

determined that epinephrine increased the rate of aqueous flow in sleeping subjects to a greater extent than it did in awake subjects; that timolol reduced the rate in awake subjects but not in sleeping subjects; and that acetazolamide reduced the rate of flow in both awake subjects and epinephrine-stimulated subjects. During sleep, acetazolamide reduced the rate of flow slightly below the basal rate, though the reduction was small and not statistically significant. In the light of these observations, these authors proposed that the diurnal fluctuation of the rate of aqueous humor flow in humans is driven by changes in the concentration of the endogenous epinephrine available to the ciliary epithelium. Moreover, because epinephrine concentration in plasma is reduced during sleep and is also lower in a supine position than in an upright position, Topper and Brubaker [168] made the interesting suggestion that endogenous epinephrine could come from the plasma to drive the diurnal variations of the rate of aqueous humor flow. However, epinephrine as well as norepinephrine have a selective secretion. Norepinephrine secretion is increased by emotional known to the individual, whereas epinephrine secretion rises in situations in which the individual meets with the unexpected [67]. It is difficult to reconcile the regular diurnal variations with the sudden rises in epinephrine concentration in plasma. Moreover, as far as we know, no data exist about the possibility of circulating endogenous epinephrine reaching the ciliary epithelium. Its high hydrophylicity sheds doubt on the theory that there is a diffusion or ultrafiltration mechanism from the blood vessels to the ciliary epithelium.

Another hypothesis supporting epinephrine could be a ciliary production of this catecholamine. However, the concentration of epinephrine in human aqueous humor seems very low: According to Cooper et al. [45], the concentration ranged from 0 to 0.1 ng/ml and was detected by Trope et al. [183] in surgical cataract patients only after retrobulbar injection containing epinephrine.

Interestingly, timolol, a potent antagonist of serotonin [110], reduced the rate of flow in awake subjects but not in sleeping subjects. The concentration of timolol necessary to cause changes in intraocular pressure is three orders of magnitude less than that required to show 50% inhibition of Na^+K^+-ATPase [102]. Indeed, timolol could decrease the aqueous humor secretion during the day by reducing serotonin stimulation of Na^+K^+-ATPase in the ciliary epithelium, thus producing a state of pseudo-sleep in the ciliary epithelium.

(2) Carboanhydrase

Since the first description by Wistrand in 1951 [193] of carbonic anhydrase activity in the ciliary processes of rabbits, this enzyme has been found in rats [114], monkeys [128], and humans [192]. Histochemical localization of carbonic anhydrase has been performed in human ciliary body [127] and found in pigmented and nonpigmented epithelium, predominantly in the basal and lateral membranes, but also in the cytoplasma. The enzyme has also been localized in the capillaries under the ciliary epithelium. In the nonpigmented epithelium, the presence of carbonic anhydrase coincided with morphological indicators of secretory activity like many infoldings and mitochondria, thin stromal tissue, and richly fenestrated capillaries [87]. Carbonic anhydrase function is still unclear. This enzyme, which catalyzes the hydration and dehydration of carbon dioxide, may contribute to the maintenance of the optimum pH for the ion transport system [43].

(3) Cyclic AMP, Ca^{2+}, and mRNA

Cyclic AMP, Ca^{2+}, and mRNA all ensure intracellular communication. Many studies have shown that these messengers play a role in the regulation of the response in hormones and drugs on the aqueous humor dynamics. Recently, Caprioli and Sears [39] proposed that the production of cyclic AMP by ciliary

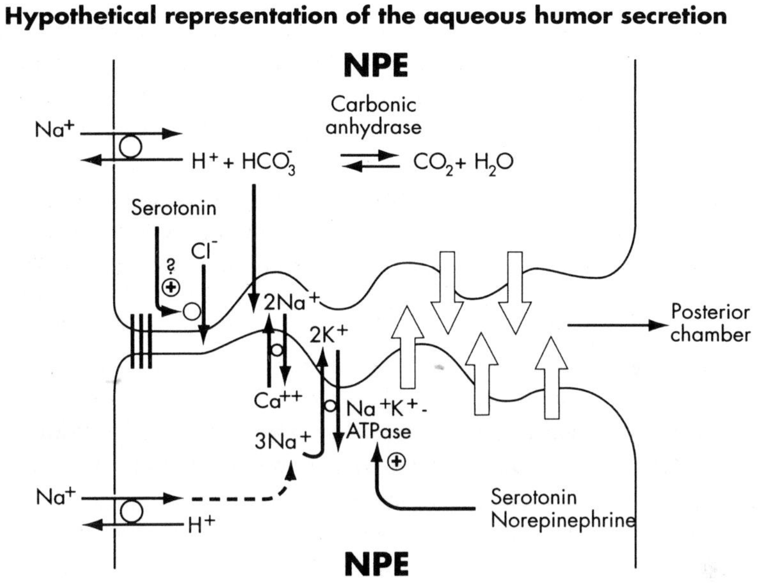

Figure 4. Hypothetical representation of the aqueous humor secretion.
The enzyme, Na^+K^+-ATPase, is predominantly located near the lateral interdigitations. Its stimulation by serotonin and noradrenaline activates the sodium-potassium pump, which determines the osmotic water flow and thus the amount of secreted aqueous humor. The chloride is probably actively secreted, and its transport, whether or not coupled with the sodium-potassium pump, could be activated by serotonin. NPE = nonpigmented ciliary epithelium.

adenylate cyclase might represent a "final common pathway" in eye-pressure regulation, and Tormay et al. [169] observed that there were at least two enzymes in the rabbit ciliary process, one regulated by calcium/calmodulin and the other by the GPT-binding regulatory protein, Gs.

To date, no information seems to be available on changes in transcription processes in relation to aqueous humor dynamics.

The hypothetical mechanism of aqueous humor secretion based on the current knowledge is summarized in Figure 4.

With regard to the regulation of aqueous humor secretion by indoleamines, the possible mechanism could be the following (Fig. 5 A and 5 B). Phospholipase C (PLC) and adenylate cyclase (AC) are not activated in light, preventing the production of N-acetyltransferase, the limiting enzyme in melatonin synthesis recently found by the author in human ciliary body [135]. Therefore, serotonin can activate Na^+K^+-ATPase, giving rise to an increase of aqueous humor formation (Fig. 5 A). On the other hand, in the dark, norepinephrine secreted by sympathetic nerve endings activates α_1 and β_2-receptors.

Thus, adenylate cyclase is activated, and c-AMP and protein phosphorylation increase, permitting the synthesis of N-acetyl-transferase. This enzyme catabolizes serotonin to N-acetylserotonin. Then, since hydroxindol-O-methyltransferase (HIOMT) and S-adenosyl-methionine (SAM) are present in excess (as observed by Malina and Martin [131]), N-acetylserotonin is catabolized to melatonin (Fig.5 B). The fact that hydroxyindol-O-methyltransferase and S-adenosyl-methionine are present in excess could explain why N-acetylserotonin was not found in the ciliary body and in aqueous humor.

3.1.4 Rate of Aqueous Humor Production

Following the initial study of Ehrlich [54] in 1882, who observed that systemically administered fluoresceine appeared in the aqueous humor of the rabbit eye, Lindner [124] as well as Amsler and Huber [2] first measured the changes in fluorescein concentration in human aqueous humor. In 1950, Goldmann [73, 74, 77] described a new method for quantifying anterior chamber fluorescence after intravenous administration of fluorescein. Goldmann found a mean aqueous flow from 1.9 to 2.2 μl/min.

Between 1965 and 1969, Holm and Krakau [91, 94, 95, 96, 97] published a series of studies using an original photographic method for volume measurements called "photogrammetric method for estimation of pupillary aqueous flow." The principle of this elegant method was the following: After instillation of pilocarpine, the pupil was made miotic, fluorescein was introduced via the cornea by iontophoresis, and the dye mixed in the aqueous by movements of the eye. Then, newly formed aqueous was seen as an uncolored "bubble" emerging from the pupil and photographed using a "slicing" or scanning method. The mean values found with this method were from 3 to 4 mm^3/min on young human volunteers and between 1 to 3 mm^3/min on glaucomas and suspected glaucoma patients [96, 97]. However, as mentioned before, pilocarpine is used to obtain the necessary miotic pupil. Furthermore, Bill [26] observed that pilocarpine reduces the uveoscleral flow of aqueous humor. Thus, Krakau wrote: "This (pilocarpine instillation) is a drawback of unknown weight since it may be that some part of the regulating range of outflow resistance is taken into account by the artificial miosis" [116].

More recently, in a study of the effect of age on aqueous humor formation in man, Brubaker et al. [38], using iontophoresis as the method of administrating fluorescein, found an increase in intraocular pressure with age of 0.093 mmHg per year and a significant decrease of anterior chamber volume with age of 1.4 μl per year. The mean anterior chamber volume was 186 ± 37 μl for all age groups. The clearance of fluorescein from the anterior chamber proceeded at a rate of approximately 1.5% of the anterior chamber volume per minute; the rate of aqueous humor formation was 2.4 µl/min. A small but statistically significant decrease in the rate of aqueous humor formation was seen for the entire group. Since aqueous humor formation is so remarkably stable with respect to aging changes, and since the intraocular pressure increases with age, according to Becker [19] it is probable that this is the consequence of the reduction of the facility of aqueous outflow. Age is not the only parameter in this regard. Elevation of the intraocular pressure involves a decrease in aqueous humor production; it is the pseudo-facility first observed by Bárány [14] and confirmed by Brubaker and Kupfer [37] and Bill [27]. A decrease of the intraocular pressure also seems to be associated with an increase in aqueous humor secretion [122].

In 1958, Ericson [56] reported that the rate of aqueous humor flow is lower during sleep, and that the suppression of flow during sleep is much greater than the change of intraocular pressure. These findings were confirmed 26 years later by Reiss et al. [148], who compared the rate of aqueous humor flow during the day, during the night in sleeping subjects, and during the night in sleep-deprived subjects. The mean rate of flow was 3.1 µl/min during the morning, 2.3 µl/min at night during sleep deprivation, and 1.6 µl/min at night during sleep. The authors suggested that a putative hormone fluctuated with the sleep cycle. Since publication of this work we have found indoleamines in human aqueous humor and indirectly observed their circadian rhythm [134, 135]. As observed previously, serotonin, a potent activator of $Na^{+}K^{+}$-ATPase, is present in high concentrations in aqueous humor during the day and is immediately catabolized into N-acetylserotonin, then to melatonin, during the night. Indoleamines are thus likely to regulate the rate of aqueous humor flow (Fig. 5 A and 5 B).

Note: During studies in 1987 measuring indoleamines in rabbit aqueous humor, I notes that the volume of the anterior chamber changed during the day. The rabbits were sampled at noon and midnight at 14-day intervals. At noon, the anterior chamber was very small, and although I successfully performed an atraumatic paracentesis in 11 rabbits under the operating microscope, this was less easily done than in humans. However, two weeks later, at midnight, I was surprised to find a very deep anterior chamber in all 11 rabbits, so that it was easy to perform the paracentesis. Roughly speaking, there is only 50% of the anterior chamber volume at noon as there is at midnight [133].

A

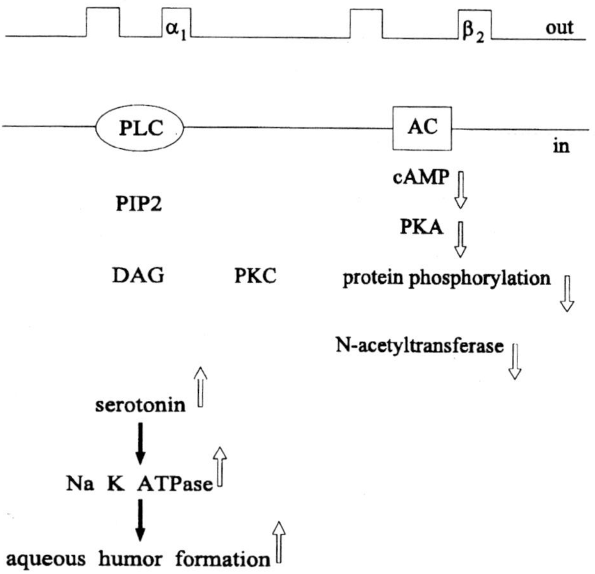

A. In light, phospholipase C (PLC) and adenylate cyclase (AC) are not activated, preventing the production of N-acetyltransferase. Thus, serotonin can activate NaK-ATPase, which gives rise to increase of aqueous humor formation.
α_1 = α_1-receptor; β_2 = β_2-receptor; cAMP = cyclic adenosine monophosphate; PIP2 = phosphatidylinositol-4',5'-b iphosphate; DAG = diacylglycerol; PKA = protein kinase A; PKC = protein kinase C.

B

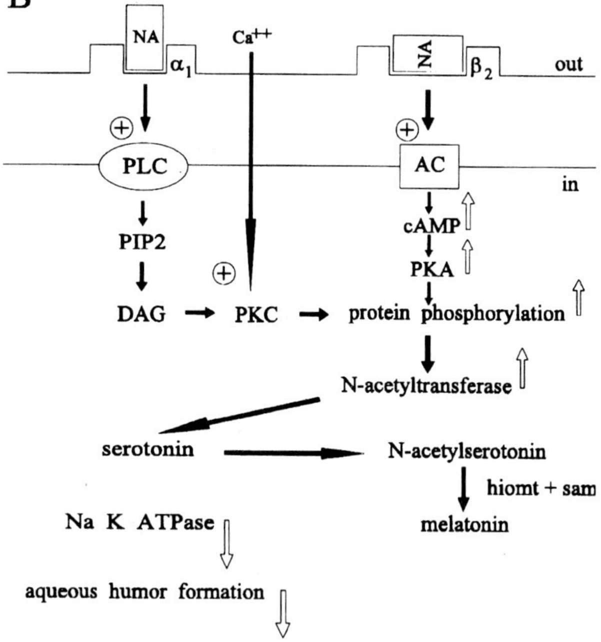

B. In the dark (or for humans during sleep), norepinephrine (NA) produced by the sympathetic nerve endings activates α_1 and β_2-receptors. Thus, AC and PLC are activated. The activation of α_1-receptors increases intracellular Ca^{2+}. Protein phosphorylation increases, permitting the synthesis of N-acetyltransferase. This enzyme catabolizes serotonin to N-acetylserotonin and, since hydroxyindole-O-methyltrans ferase (HIOMT) and S-adenosyl-L-methionine (SAM) are present in excess, to melatonin. The NaK-ATPase is no longer stimulated and the aqueous humor formation decreases.

Figure 5. Possible regulation of aqueous humor formation in human non-pigmented ciliary epithelium.

3.2 Evacuation Through the Outflow System

The evacuation of the aqueous humor, i. e., outflow, depends on the resistance in two different systems – a canalicular system and a noncanalicular system localized anterior and posterior to the scleral spur, respectively.

From a functional point of view, the canalicular system can be divided into two parts separated by the inner wall of Schlemm's canal. The anterior part of the trabecular meshwork is located between the anterior chamber and the inner wall of Schlemm's canal, and the second part consists of Schlemm's canal, the intrascleral channels, and the episcleral and conjunctival veins.

The noncanalicular system consists of the posterior part of the uveal trabecular meshwork, the interstitial spaces between the fibers of the ciliary muscle, and the supraciliary and suprachoroidal spaces. From there, the aqueous passes through the sclera via spaces between the collagen fibrils and through loose connective tissue along the nerves and blood vessels transfixing the sclera [33].

3.2.1 Canalicular System

For Goldmann [72, 73], Weekers [185, 186], and Bárány [18], the resistance to aqueous outflow is localized in the trabecular meshwork. According to Goldmann [72], in humans 75% of the resistance is induced by this structure, with 25% occurring beyond Schlemm's canal. These findings were later confirmed by Grant [79], who removed the trabecular meshwork of enucleated human eyes previously trephined and then made measurements of facility of outflow by perfusion under direct view with a binocular dissecting microscope and at a magnification of 40×. Grant found that the trabecular meshwork is responsible for approximately 75% of the total resistance to outflow of fluid from the anterior chamber. On this basis, he proposed trabeculotomy and trabeculectomy as surgical therapies for open-angle glaucoma. These studies encouraged Sugar to perform the first trabeculectomies on humans, the results of which were published in 1961 [164].

If 75% of the outflow resistance is located in the trabecular meshwork, the remaining 25% must be attributed to Schlemm's canal as well as other channels thereafter, the venous system, and the noncanalicular outflow system.

(1) Trabecular Meshwork and Glycosaminoglycans (formerly "mucopolysaccharides")

In 1956, Brini [34], using histochemical techniques, observed a hyaluronidase-like substance in the human trabecular meshwork. Ashton [10], François et al.

[62], Zimmermann [196], and Berggren et al. [21] confirmed this observation. These authors found more mucopolysaccharide in part of the trabecular adjacent to the inner wall of Schlemm's canal. Fine [60] designated this region "juxtacanalicular tissue." Later, it was established that mucopolysaccharides or glycosaminoglycans occur in the form of hyaluronic acid, chondroitin sulfate, and dermatan sulfate [138]. Using ruthenium-red staining to identify glycosaminoglycans with electron microscopy in the cat, Richardson [149] localized these constituents of the extracellular matrix on the surfaces of the endothelial cells in the trabecular meshwork and aqueous plexus, within their basal laminae, and in the amorphous tissue of the trabecular beams and tissue adjacent to the aqueous plexus. The location of glycosaminoglycans in the juxtacanalicular meshwork of the cat seems very similar to that found in monkey and humans in other studies [8, 84, 88, 138]. In addition to these morphological studies, Knepper et al. [111] undertook biochemical analyses of glycosaminoglycans in rabbit aqueous outflow pathway and iris-ciliary body, and found the following glycosaminoglycans: hyaluronic acid, keratan sulfate and hybrid dermatan sulfate-chondroiton sulfate. In another study [112], the same authors observed that *Streptomyces hyaluronidase* is more effective than testicular hyaluronidase in decreasing aqueous outflow resistance, and that hyaluronic acid is an important glycosaminoglycan contributor to aqueous outflow resistance in the normal rabbit eye.

These histochemical and biochemical observations support and specify the physiological findings of Bárány [12, 13, 15, 16, 17, 18], who has shown by animal experimentation that the removal of hyaluronic acid by injection of hyaluronidase into the anterior chamber might lower the resistance to aqueous outflow by about 50%. On the other hand, he found that resistance rose when he perfused the eye with high-molecular hyaluronic acid. The latter is today very well-known in human cataract surgery. Indeed, if hyaluronic acid is used during cataract operation and left in the eye, a high intraocular pressure increase can be observed for some days.

The physiological role of the mucopolysaccharides that constituted the fundamental substance of the trabecular meshwork was already understood by Bárány [12, 13, 16] and Amsler [3, 5]. Indeed, Amsler et al. [3, 5] spoke of the spongy aspect of the trabecular meshwork on freshly enucleated eyes and attributed this aspect to the mucopolysaccharides partly responsible for the resistance to outflow in the trabecular meshwork. The hydration of the trabecular meshwork can be explained by the osmotic forces exerted by the glycosaminoglycans.

Hyaluronic acid is found in aqueous humor [118, 119, 137] and trabecular meshwork. As far as we know, there are no publications dealing the origin of the aqueous hyaluronic acid and the possibility of its production in ciliary epithelium. However, in the trabecular meshwork, hyaluronic acid is produced by tissue culture of primate trabecular cells [154], and hyaluronic acid and fibronectin are produced by cultured human trabecular cells [145, 194]. On the other hand, endogenous hyaluronidase has been isolated in cultured human trabecular cells [197]. The coexistence of hyaluronic acid and hyaluronidase in the same structure permits the hypothesis that hyaluronidase might participate in the regulation of the resistance of the trabecular meshwork. To what extent these observations – derived from tissue cultures of trabecular meshwork cells – can be useful remains unanswered, since these cells can quickly adapt their morphology to a culture environment, and since the adult human meshwork contains a significant population of nontrabecular cells [79].

François et al. [63] proposed an interesting explanation for the pathogenesis of corticosteroid glaucoma, establishing a correlation between corticosteroid and glycosaminoglycans metabolism:

> "The non-depolymerised [sic] mucopolysaccharides of the anterior chamber angle can become hydrated. This biological oedema can obstruct the trabeculae, but the physiological liberation of catabolic enzymes from the lysosomes depolymerises the mucopolysaccharides and prevents this obstruction. This is, on the contrary, facilitated by the corticosteroids, which reinforce the lysosomal membranes and impede the liberation of the catabolic enzymes."

In a series of experiments, Southren et al. [163] and Weinstein et al. [189] observed that cells cultured from specimens obtained by trabeculectomy from patients with primary open-angle glaucoma showed an altered pattern of cortisol metabolism leading to the accumulation of both 5-α and 5-β-dihydrocortisol, intermediates not found in similar trabecular cells derived from patients without primary open-angle glaucoma. Assays of cortisol-metabolizing enzymes in homogenates of trabecular cells of patients with primary open-angle glaucoma indicated that the accumulation of dihydrocortisol results from alterations in two enzymes, an increase in cortisol-δ-4-reductase, and a decrease in 3-oxydoreductase. On the other hand, 5-β-hydroxycortisol, which accumulated abnormally in cultured cells of trabeculum from patients with primary open-angle glaucoma [162], was found to potentiate glucocorticoid activity [188].

These pathological findings in trabecular cells of patients with primary open-angle glaucoma might help us to understand the possible role of corticoid metabolism in these cells as well as the correlation to the changes in outflow facility. In this connection, glucocorticoid receptors have been observed in the membrane of the human trabecular cells [93, 187].

Finally, an attempt was made experimentally to bind again the possible effect of corticoids on trabecular cells and the incorporation of precursors of certain glycosaminoglycans [92].

Recently, Tripathi et al. [170] observed by histochemical-electronmicroscopic method that sialic acid moieties, already found in aqueous humor and vitreous, are present in trabecular meshwork. Tripathi et al. [170] observed in the juxtacanalicular tissue zone a random distribution of the extracellular elements, and an almost continuous coat was present around the cell surfaces. Quantitatively, there was an increase in sialic acid moieties in the trabecular meshwork of eyes with primary open-angle glaucoma. Since the sialic acid moieties are implicated in increasing intrinsic viscosity of all glycoproteins, they might contribute to the increased resistance to aqueous outflow.

Using a theoretical model, about 80% of the resistance of the trabecular meshwork to aqueous humor outflow were found to be localized in the subendothelial region of the juxtacanalicular meshwork; this resistance is induced by the glycosaminoglycans [57, 158].

(2) Inner-Wall Endothelium of Schlemm's Canal

Although Feeney and Wissig [59] were presumably the first to observe the transcellular transport in the inner wall or trabecular wall of Schlemm's canal using electron-dense tracer, the main contribution was from Tripathi [171, 172, 173, 174, 175, 176], who proposed a cyclical sequence of events in the formation of vacuolar transcellular channels that constitute a dynamic system of pores as well as the mechanism of bulk outflow of the aqueous humor across the mesothelial barrier of Schlemm's canal. According to Tripathi [171], the bulk outflow of aqueous humor takes place down a pressure gradient from the trabecular meshwork into Schlemm's canal via such vacuolar transcellular channels which act as one-way valves. In several works on the pressure-induced changes in the ultrastructure of the endothelium lining Schlemm's canal, Grierson and Lee [81, 82, 83] observed that significant modifications occurred at the fine structural level in the pinosomes, micropinosomes, giant vacuoles, and the nonvacuolar transcellular channels. They observed that giant vacuoles were absent when the intraocular pressure was 0 mmHg, and that their number lay between 22 and 30 mmHg, decreasing with higher pressure. In addition, they found no morphological evidence to indicate that energy consumption or protein production was necessary to increase the vacuole population in the endothelium, thus reinforcing Tripathi's hypothesis that the vacuolization process results from a distortion of the endothelial cell, a response to hydrostatic pressure. Moreover, Grierson et al. [81, 82, 83] postulated that the endothelial pliability probably depends on cytoplasmic microfilaments, already described in Schlemm's canal inner wall endothelium and juxtacanalicular meshwork in the monkey [100], which were found to be in contact with the vacuole membrane. These findings can be correlated with the intracameral perfusion experiments of Kaufman and Bárány [103, 104], who observed that perfusion of cytochalasin B (known to disrupt contractile microfilaments [190]) decreased resistance to outflow by about 75%. The cytochalasin effect was apparent in less than 20 minutes and was largely reversible over a few hours. Structural changes in the anterior ocular segment, particularly in the trabecular meshwork, after cytochalasin B intracameral perfusion were subsequently described [165]. Using different monkey species and perfusion techniques, Johnstone et al. [101] and Kaufman et al. [105] found similar concentration-dependent morphologic effects of cytochalasin B in the aqueous outflow system. Moreover, in the same study, Kaufman et al. determined that cytochalasin D was about 25 times more potent than cytochalasin B. Intracameral perfusion with ethylenediaminetetraacetic acid (EDTA) [23, 106, 184], and (ethyleneglycol-bis-beta-aminoethylether) -N-N'-tetraacetic acid (EGTA) produced a very large increase in gross outflow facility, and electron-microscopic studies showed marked ruptures in the inner wall of Schlemm's canal, a wash-out of extracellular material, and other alterations of the trabecular meshwork.

In scanning electron-microscopic studies of the human trabecular meshwork and Schlemm's canal, Bill and Svedbergh [25] found that 10% of the total trabecular resistance resided in the inner wall endothelium of Schlemm's canal; Moseley et al. [141], using a mathematical modelling of aqueous humor outflow from the eye through the pores in the endothelial lining of Schlemm's canal, found 18%.

3.2.2 Uveoscleral Outflow or Noncanalicular System

Troncoso [177, 178, 179, 180, 181, 182] was probably the first to think that the aqueous humor could leave the anterior chamber of the eye by two different pathways, the canalicular one and the uveoscleral one. Later, Kiss [109], Henderson [90], and Schreck [156] came to the same conclusion. However, the merit of the discovery probably belongs to Schreck in 1949, who observed the tracer in the canalicular system and also in the uveal meshwork after injecting a colorant in the anterior chamber five minutes before enucleation. Between 1965 and 1971, Bill et al. [22, 24, 26, 30, 31] performed a series of physiological experiments, demonstrating in vervet and cynomolgus monkeys as well as humans that the uveoscleral drainage plays an important role in the drainage of aqueous humor. It was observed in the human eye [24] that between 4 and

14% of the aqueous humor passes from the anterior chamber into the anterior uvea, and from there into the suprachoroid and out of the eye, through perivascular spaces as well as diffusely through the scleral tissue. It was also observed that in eyes treated with atropine uveoscleral flow was 4–27% of the total outflow, but in the pilocarpine-treated eyes only 0–3%.

3.3 Normal Intraocular Pressure

3.3.1 Method of Measurement

The principle of the method is based on the relationship between the intraocular pressure and the force deriving from external deformation of the cornea. The deformation can be obtained by indentation, for example, with the Schiøtz tonometer [155] or by applanation, for example, with the Maklakoff [130] and Goldmann tonometers [75]. Although the pressure is measured on the external cornea, the used term is "intraocular pressure."

Since its introduction in 1954, the Goldmann applanation tonometer has become by far the tonometer most used among ophthalmologists.

The Goldmann tonometer principle is based on the perspicacious article on ophthalmotonometric theory published in 1885 by Imbert [99]. This principle, known as the Imbert-Fick law, was improved by Goldmann and Schmidt [71], who adapted the formula and took into account the fact that the cornea is a membrane of finite thickness and stiffness, and that the liquid between the cornea and the flattening device develops capillary forces. Goldmann found that, with a diameter of the flattened area of 3 and 3.5 mm, the elastic and capillary forces balance each other out in normal human cornea, and that, with such a diameter of flattened cornea, the displaced volume was only 0.5 mm^3, considerably less than the 15–20 mm^3 with a Schiøtz tonometer [76]. Two other applanation tonometers are currently in use, the Perkins applanation tonometer and the Draeger applanation tonometer, both of which are hand-held and use the Goldmann applanation tonometric principle.

Recently, three different tonometers, the Schiøtz, the Perkins, and the Tono-Pen, a electronic applanation tonometer, were compared with regard to their increasing intraocular effect on eye-bank eyes. Perkins tonometry produced a mean intraocular pressure increase of 0.7 mmHg, the Tono-Pen tonometry 12.1 mmHg, and the Schiøtz tonometry 16.5 mmHg [191].

The Goldmann applanation tonometer is a very accurate, easily calibrated measuring instrument. Although these qualities have been questioned by Arciniegas et al. [7], it remains the most used tonometer and the standard on which other tonometers are measured.

The sources of error deriving from the use of the Goldmann tonometer are without clinical importance when the cornea is normal, the anterior chamber is present, and the instrument is used properly [142].

3.3.2 Normal Intraocular Pressure in Infants and Children

Intraocular pressure increases with age. In the only reported study on premature infants [35], intraocular pressure was measured with the Schiøtz tonometer, the mean intraocular pressure in 59 infants being 24.5 mmHg with a range of 6.5 to 33 mmHg. The indentation method used, and the large dispersion of the data demonstrate the difficulty in performing this measurement in these children.

(1) In Newborns under Topical Anesthesia

In normal-term newborns under topical anesthesia, the measurements made with indentation tonometry show very large dispersion of values, between 10.2 and 56 mmHg [51, 69, 98].

In the only study performed in newborns with topical anesthesia and applanation tonometry, the mean intraocular pressure was 11.4 ± 2.4 mmHg (range 6 to 17) [146].

(2) In Newborns Under General Anesthesia

In normal-term newborns under general anesthesia, intraocular pressure was measured with the Schiøtz tonometer and Draeger hand-held tonometer. While the intraocular pressure was between 14.7 and 22.2 mmHg in newborns [78, 115] with the Schiøtz tonometer, the intraocular pressure with the hand-held Draeger applanation tonometer was between 7 and 20 mmHg, with an average of 13.4 mmHg [78].

(3) In Infants a Few Days Old up to 5 Years under General Anesthesia

In children of a few days up to 5 years of age, the mean values with applanation tonometry vary between 7.8 and 11.7 mmHg [52, 70, 86, 152]. Goethals and Missotten [70] measured intraocular pressure in 44 children between 4 months and 5 years under halothane anesthesia using the Perkins hand-held applanometer. The mean intraocular pressure was 7.8 mmHg for children between 4 months to 1 year, increasing 1 mmHg more each year up to 5 years of age, where it was 11.7 mmHg.

3.3.3 Ocular Pressure Effect of Anesthetics

Whereas topical anesthesia of the cornea with oxybuprocaine – the most widely used anesthetic – has no observable effect on the intraocular pressure [123], general anesthesia, particularly with halothane (Fluothane), the most widely used substance, is controversial. Indeed, whereas several animal and human studies have claimed that general anesthesia usually produces lower intraocular pressure [117, 147, 159], studies performed in children do not confirm this view, finding no intraocular pressure value changes under general anesthesia at all [11, 52, 86, 157]. The author has observed that the type tonometer used has more influence than the type of anesthetic drug used, and whether halothane has a tensional effect or not, is more hypotensive.

However, certain substances, such as ketamine, an arylcycloalkylamine frequently used for brief anesthesia in children, are known to increase intraocular pressure [46]. In a comparative study of tensional effects of halothane and ketamine in a group of 13 children between 11 and 14 years of age who were anesthetized a first time with halothane and a second time with ketamine, Maddox and Kielhar [129], using a Schiøtz tonometer, measured a mean intraocular pressure of 12.4 mmHg under halothane and 16.7 mmHg under ketamine.

Other substances, such as succinylcholine [47], used as a myorelaxant to facilitate endotracheal intubation, produce a transitory increased in intraocular pressure up to 18 mmHg more than the baseline pressure. This tensional response varies according to the type of drug association [68, 121, 166] and occurs between the 10th and the 40th second after intravenous injection. This hypertensional transitory effect must be considered when intubating a patient with an ocular performation or wound dehiscence. Although a recent experimental study performed in cat eyes found that the administration of succinylcholine did not give rise to loss of eye content [139], clinical experience in humans shows that this complication was possible following a concomitant contraction of rectus muscles [6, 58, 140].

Nitrous oxide (laughing gas) mixed with oxygen as used in general anesthesia, like chloral [147], produces an elevation of intraocular pressure [159].

Finally, administration of oxygen decreases intraocular pressure [65], and carbon dioxide increases it [108, 144, 153].

3.3.4 Normal Intraocular Pressure in Adults and the Elderly

Intraocular pressure results from the balance between inflow and outflow. As long as the ocular tonus remains optimal for the conservation of the visual function, intraocular pressure can be considered normal.

Mean normal intraocular pressure is usually reported by combining all age groups and taking one measurement with no regard to time of day [9, 125, 151]. In four studies using applanation tonometry and reporting intraocular pressure distribution in the general population [9, 125, 143, 151], the intraocular pressure mean values were between 15 and 17 mmHg. The mean age of groups in three of the studies mentioned [9, 125, 151] was greater than 47 years. In the Framingham Eye Study, the mean age of the participants was 65 years (range 52 to 85), the mean intraocular pressure 16.5 mmHg [120].

However, intraocular pressure increases with age, this increase probably being related to reduced facility of aqueous outflow [19], since aqueous humor production slowly decreases with age by –0.006 µl/min/year, viz. about 20% in the course a lifetime [38]. Moreover, intraocular pressure fluctuates diurnally from 3 mmHg to 6 mmHg [50]. Therefore, "normal" intraocular pressure should be reported as the average of several measurements at different times of the day in a homogeneous, normal group, that is, a group of young, healthy adults.

In order to determine the normal intraocular pressure of such a group, Martin [136] measured the intraocular pressure in 24 healthy caucasian volunteers aged 23–39 years (average 28 years ± 4 SD) with no history of ocular disease or refractive error greater than ± 4 diopters. All subjects were resident physicians in the University Eye Clinic at either Lausanne or Basel. Each subject underwent an ophthalmological examination including visual acuity, biomicroscopy, Goldmann or automated perimetry, tonometry,and fundus in mydriasis. Intraocular pressure was measured in 12 subjects (Group 1) every hour between 8 a. m. and 10 p. m., resulting in a total of 360 measurements (12 subjects × 2 eyes × 15 measurements on each eye). In Group 2 (also 12 subjects), intraocular pressure was measured at 8 a. m., 11 a. m., 2 p. m., and 5 p. m., resulting in 96 measurements (12 subjects × 2 eyes × 4 measurements). Two calibrated Goldmann applanation tonometers (model T 900 Haag-Streit, Bern, Switzerland) were used, one for Group 1 and the other for Group 2. The same biprism was used for all measurements in Group 1 and another biprism for Group 2; the biprism was disinfected for each subject. The measurements were taken first for the right eye, then for the left eye, then repeated in the same order. If the second measurement on the right eye was identical to that of the first measurement, a third measurement was not performed. Otherwise, a third measurement was performed on both sides, the average of the three consecutive readings being noted down. By comparison, in the Framingham Eye Study the average of three measurements was systematically calculated, though with two different methods: applanation tonometry in the majority of the cases and Schiøtz tonometry in some cases [120].

Table 1. Mean intraocular pressure measured hourly between 8 a.m., and 10 p.m. (Group 1).

Subjects			Intraocular pressure (mm Hg)			
			Right eye		Left eye	
	Sex	Age	Mean*	SD	Mean*	SD
1	F	24	11.3	±1.2	10.9	±1.2
2	F	26	12.0	±2.1	13.1	±1.5
3	F	24	11.3	±1.6	10.9	±1.4
4	M	26	11.6	±1.5	12.3	±1.1
5	M	26	10.9	±1.5	10.2	±1.2
6	M	26	7.5	±1.2	7.6	±0.9
7	M	25	10.5	±1.4	10.5	±1.4
8	M	23	8.9	±1.2	8.4	±1.2
9	M	25	10.5	±1.0	12.4	±1.2
10	M	24	11.9	±1.3	11.7	±1.3
11	M	27	11.1	±1.8	11.7	±1.6
12	M	28	14.0	±1.9	13.9	±2.1

* Mean intraocular pressure measured hourly between 8 a. m., and 10 p. m., i. e., 15 measurements in each eye. SD = standard deviation.

Table 2. Mean intraocular pressure measured at 8 a.m., 11 a.m., 2 p.m., and 5 p.m. (Group 2).

Subjects			Intraocular pressure (mm Hg)			
			Right eye		Left eye	
	Sex	Age	Mean*	SD	Mean*	SD
1	F	32	11.0	±1.8	11.5	±1.9
2	F	25	10.2	±1.7	11.5	±1.3
3	F	30	14.2	±1.7	15.2	±2.0
4	F	34	12.0	±1.8	11.7	±1.0
5	M	28	11.5	±0.6	11.7	±0.9
6	M	25	11.5	±1.9	11.7	±1.7
7	M	27	14.5	±1.3	13.7	±0.5
8	M	34	15.0	±2.1	14.2	±2.2
9	M	34	11.2	±1.7	11.2	±1.5
10	M	39	9.5	±1.0	10.0	±0.0
11	M	29	12.7	±1.5	13.0	±0.8
12	M	30	13.2	±0.9	13.7	±1.2

* Mean intraocular pressure measured at 8 a. m., 11 a. m., 2 p. m., and 5 p. m., i. e., 4 measurements in each eye. SD = standard deviation.

Table 1 gives the mean intraocular pressure in Group 1, Table 2 that of Group 2. Table 3 gives the mean intraocular pressure in the two groups.

The groups differ in the lowest intraocular pressures found after 5 p. m. These results show an intraocular pressure of 26.7% lower in Group 1 and 18.0% lower in Group 2 than the 15 mmHg generally considered to be normal intraocular pressure. This important difference can be explained in that the

Table 3. Mean intraocular pressure.

Eyes (n = 48)	Mean intraocular pressure (mm Hg)	
	Group 1 (360 measurements)*	Group 2 (96 measurements)**
Right eyes (n = 24)	10.9 ± 1.6 SD	12.2 ± 1.7 SD
Left eyes (n = 24)	11.1 ± 1.8 SD	12.4 ± 1.5 SD
Mean values (n = 48)	11.0 ± 1.7 SD	12.3 ± 1.6 SD

* 12 subjects, 24 eyes, and 15 measurements per eye.
** 12 subjects, 24 eyes, and 4 measurements per eye.

value of 15 mmHg is based on mass screening, which does not consider intraocular pressure to be a variable but a constant. Further, when the same principles are applied to this study and only a single morning measurement is considered, the mean intraocular pressure is 13.3 mmHg ± 2.7 SD in Group 1, 2.2 mmHg higher than the mean. The average age in Group 1 (25 years ± 1.4 SD) probably explains the remaining difference between the 13.3 and the 15 mmHg considered to be mean normal value.

As mentioned above, by definition the normal intraocular pressure allows optimal function of the eye. Now, an 11-year follow-up study suggests that an intraocular pressure over 17 mmHg is sufficient to make glaucomatous damage progress in half of the patients with primary open-angle glaucoma [132]. Although factors other than pressure are involved in glaucoma disease, it is difficult to consider the mean intraocular pressure of 17.18 mmHg found in more than 4,500 "normal" subjects in one study already cited [125] to be normal intraocular pressure. The author is in agreement with a number of others [113, 160] who think that the explanation leads to an overlapping of intraocular pressure distributions within nonglaucoma and glaucoma populations.

Since intraocular pressure is indeed a variable, its normal value can only be the *average* of its various values throughout the day. We propose that, like other biological parameters, normal intraocular pressure be based on measurements from healthy, homogeneous groups.

In conclusion, the author suggests that normal mean intraocular pressure in adults measured during the day with the Goldmann applanation tonometer is 12±3 mmHg and increases of about 1 mmHg each decade between the ages of 40 and 80.

References

1. Adler FH. The Aqueous. In Adler FH (ed.) Physiology of the Eye. Clinical Application. St-Louis: The C.V. Mosby Company 1950, p. 107.
2. Amsler M, Huber A. Methodik und erste klinische Ergebnisse einer Funktionprüfung der Blut-Kammerwasser-Schranke. Ophthalmologica 1946; 111:155–176.
3. Amsler M, Verrey F, Huber A. L'humeur aqueuse tensionnelle et ses problèmes rhéologiques. In Amsler M, Verrey F, Huber A (eds.) L'Humeur aqueuse et ses fonctions. Paris: Masson, 1955, pp. 36 and 56.
4. Amsler M, Verrey F, Huber A. Production de l'humeur aqueuse. In Amsler M, Verrey F, Huber A (eds.) L'humeur aqueuse et ses fonctions. Paris: Masson, 1955, pp. 123–124.
5. Amsler M. Die Autopsie des Auges. Ber Dtsch Ophthalmol Ges 1950; 56:100–112.
6. Anderson DR. Discussion, pp. 474–475; cited in Joshi C, Bruce DL: Thiopental and succinylcholine: Action on intraocular pressure. Anesth Analg 1975; 54:471–475.
7. Arciniegas A, Amaya LE, Hernàndez LM. Physical factors that influence the measurement of the intraocular pressure with Goldmann's tonometer. New Trends Ophthalmol 1986; 1:170–200.
8. Armaly MF, Wang Y. Demonstration of acid mucopoly-saccharides in the trabecular meshwork of the rhesus monkey. Invest Ophthalmol 1975; 14:507–516.
9. Armaly MF. On the distribution of applanation pressure. I. Statistical features and effect of age, sex, and family history of glaucoma. Arch Ophthalmol 1965; 73:11–18.
10. Ashton N, Brini A, Smith R. Anatomical studies of the trabecular meshwork of the normal human eye. Brit J Ophthalmol 1956; 40:257–282.
11. Ausinsch B, Graves SA, Munson ES, Levy NS. Intraocular pressures in children during isoflurane and halothane anesthesia. Anesthesiology 1975; 42:167–172.
12. Bárány EH, Scotchbrook S. Influence of testicular hyaluronidase on the resistance to flow through the angle of the the anterior chamber. Acta Physiol Scand 1954; 30:240–248.
13. Bárány EH, Woodin AM. Hyaluronic acid and hyaluronidase in the aqueous humour and the angle of the anterior chamber. Acta Physiol Scand 1955; 33:257–290.
14. Bárány EH. A mathematical formulation of intraocular pressure as dependant on secretion, ultrafiltration, bulk outflow, and osmotic reabsorption of fluid. Invest Ophthalmol 1963; 2:584–590.
15. Bárány EH. In vitro studies of the resistance to flow through the angle of the anterior chamber. Acta Soc Med Uppsala 1954; 59:260–276.
16. Bárány EH. Physiologic and pharmacologic factors influencing the resistance to aqueous outflow. In Newell FW (ed.), Glaucoma. Trans Int Conf, Princeton, Josiah Macy, Jr. Foundation, 1955; 123–221.
17. Bárány EH. The action of different kinds of hyaluronidase on the resistance to flow through the angle of anterior chamber. Acta Ophthalmol 1956; 34:397–403.
18. Bárány E. Experimental studies on aqueous outflow. Acta XVII Concil Ophthalmol (1954), vol. 3. Montreal-New York: University of Toronto Press. 1954, p. 1546.
19. Becker B. The decline in aqueous secretion and outflow facility with age. Am J Ophthalmol 1958; 46:731–736.
20. Becker B. Vanadate and aqueous humor dynamics. Proctor Lecture. Invest Ophthalmol Vis Sci 1980; 19:1156–1165.

21. Berggren L, Vrabec F. Demonstration of a coating substance in the trabecular meshwork of the eye and its decrease after perfusion experiments with different kinds of hyaluronidase. Am J Ophthalmol 1957; 44:200–208.

22. Bill A, Hellsing K. Production and drainage of aqueous humor in the cynomolgus monkey (Macaca irus). Invest Ophthalmol 1965; 4:920–926.

23. Bill A, Lütjen-Drecoll E, Svedbergh B. Effects of intra-cameral Na2EDTA and EGTA on aqueous outflow routes in the monkey eye. Invest Ophthalmol Vis Sci 1980; 19:492–504.

24. Bill A, Phillips CI. Uveoscleral drainage of aqueous humor in human eyes. Exp Eye Res 1971; 12:275–281.

25. Bill A, Svedbergh B. Scanning electron microscopic studies of the trabecular meshwork and the canal of Schlemm. An attempt to localize the main resistance to outflow of aqueous humor in man. Acta Ophthalmol 1972; 50:295–320.

26. Bill A, Wålhinder PE. The effect of pilocarpine on the dynamics of aqueous humor in a primate (Macaca irus). Invest Ophthalmol 1966; 5:170–175.

27. Bill A, Bárány EH. Gross facility, facility of conventional routes, and pseudofacility of aqueous humor outflow in the cynomolgus monkey. Arch Ophthalmol 1966; 75:665–673.

28. Bill A. Aspects on suppressibility of aqueous humor formation. Doc Ophthalmol 1969; 26:73–80.

29. Bill A. Blood circulation and fluid dynamics in the eye. Physiol Rev 1975; 55:383–417.

30. Bill A. Effects of atropine on aqueous humor dynamics in the Vervet monkey (Cercopithecus ethiops). Exp Eye Res 1969; 8:284–291.

31. Bill A. The aqueous humor drainage mechanism in the cynomolgus monkey (Macaca irus) with evidence for unconventional routes. Invest Ophthalmol 1965; 4:911–919.

32. Bill A. The role of ciliary blood flow and ultrafiltration in aqueous humor formation. Exp Eye Res 1973; 16:287–298.

33. Bill A. Basic physiology of the drainage of aqueous humor. Exp Eye Res 1977; 25 (Suppl):291–304.

34. Brini MA. Mise en évidence, à l'aide de techniques histochimiques, d'une substance sensible à l'hyaluronidase dans le trabéculum de l'oeil humain. Bull Soc Ophthal Paris 1956; 2:256–264.

35. Brockhurst RJ. The intraocular pressure of premature infants. Am J Ophthalmol 1955; 39:808–811.

36. Brodwall J, Fischbarg J. The hydraulic conductivity of rabbit ciliary epithelium in vitro. Exp Eye Res 1982; 34:121–129.

37. Brubaker RF, Kupfer C. Determination of pseudofacility in the eye of the rhesus monkey. Arch Ophthalmol 1966; 75:693–697.

38. Brubaker RF, Nagataki S, Townsend DJ, Burns RR, Higgins RG, Wentworth W. The effect of age on aqueous formation in man. Ophthalmology 1981; 88:283–287.

39. Caprioli J, Sears ML. The adenylate cyclase receptor complex and aqueous humor formation. Yale J Biol Med 1984; 57:283–300.

40. Cheng LC, Rogus EM, Zierler K. Catechol, astructural requirement for $Na^{+}K^{+}$-ATPase stimulation in rat skeletal muscle membrane. Biochim Biophys Acta 1977; 464:338–346.

41. Coffee RG, Hadden JW, Hadden EM, Middleton E Jr. Stimulation of ATPase by norepinephrine: an α-adrenergic receptor mechanism. Abstract. Federation Proc 1971; 30: 497.

42. Cole DF. Location of ouabain-sensitive adenosine triphosphate in ciliary epithelium. Exp Eye Res 1964; 3:72–75.

43. Cole DF. Secretion of the aqueous humor. Exp Eye Res 1977; 25 (Suppl):161–176.

44. Cole DF. Ocular Fluids. In Davson H (ed.) The Eye, vol. 1A, Vegetative Physiology and Biochemistry. Orlando: Academic Press, 1984, pp. 269–390.

45. Cooper RL, Constable IJ, Davidson L. Aqueous humor catecholamines. Curr Eye Res 1984; 3:809–813.

46. Corssen G, Hoy JE. A new parenteral anesthetic-C1–581:Its effect on intraocular pressure. J Pediatr Ophthalmol 1967; 4:20–23.

47. Craythorne NWB, Rottenstein HS, Dripps, RD. The effect of succinylcholine on intraocular pressure in adults, infants and children during general anesthesia. Anesthesiology 1960; 21:59–63.

48. Davson H, Luck, CP. A comparative study of the total carbon dioxyde in the ocular fluids, cerebrospinal fluid, and plasma of some mammalian species. J Physiol 1957; 132:454–464.

49. Davson H, Spaziani E. The fate of substances injected into the anterior chamber of the eye. J Physiol 1960; 151:202–215.

50. De Venecia G, Davis MD. Diurnal variation of intraocular pressure in the normal eye. Arch Ophthalmol 1963; 69:752–757.

51. Dolcet L. Tension ocular del risien nacido. Arch Soc Oftalmol Hisp Am 1952; 12: 1057–1063.

52. Dominguez A, Baños MS, Alvarez MG, Contra GF, Quintela FB. Intraocular pressure measurement in infants under general anesthesia. Am J Ophthalmol 1974; 78:110–116.

53. Duke-Elder S. The formation of the aqueous humour. In Duke-Elder D (ed.) System of Ophthalmology, vol. 4. The Physiology of the Eye and of Vision. London: Henry Kimpton, 1968, pp. 186–187.

54. Ehrlich P. Ueber provocirte Fluorescenzerscheinungen am Auge. Dtsch Med Wochenschr 1882; 8:35–37.

55. Eisen HN, Fields B, Goldberg AL, Karnovsky ML, Kennedy, EP. Active transport of sodium and potassium ions. The New Eng J of Med 1980; 302:777–783.

56. Ericson LA. Twenty-four hourly variations in the inflow of the aqueous humor. Acta Ophthalmol 1958; 36:381–385.

57. Ethier CR, Kamm RD, Palaszewski BA, Johnson MC, Richardson TM. Calculations of flow resistance in the juxtacanlicular meshwork. Invest Ophthalmol Vis Sci 1986; 27:1741–1750.

58. Evans LS. Letter to the editor. Ophthalmology 1991; 98:1608.

59. Feeney L, Wissig S. Outflow studies using an electron dense tracer. Trans Am Acad Ophthalmol Otol 1966; 70:791–798.

60. Fine BS. Observations on the drainage angle in man and rhesus monkey: a concept of the pathogenesis of chronic simple glaucoma. A light and electron microscopic study. Invest Ophthalmol 1964; 3:609–646.

61. Flammer J, Gasser P, Shaw S, Guthauser U, Weidmann R. Intraokuläre Katecholaminkonzentrationen. Klin Mbl Augenheilk 1986; 188:503–504.

62. François J, Neetens A, Collette JM. Microradiographic study of the influence of hyaluronidase on the permeability of the inner wall of Schlemm's canal. Am J Ophthalmol 1956; 41:651–657.

63. François J, Victoria-Troncoso V. Corticosteroid glaucoma. Ophthalmologica 1977; 174:195–209.

64. Friedenwald JS. The formation of the intraocular fluid. Am J Ophthalmol 1949; 32:9–27.

65. Gallin-Cohen PF, Podos SM, Yablonski ME. Oxygen lowers intraocular pressure. Invest Ophthalmol Vis Sci 1980; 19:43–48.

66. Ganong WF. Physiologic Principles. In Ganong WF (ed.) Review of Medical Physiology, 12th ed. Los Altos: Lange Medical Publications, 1985; 19–20.

67. Ganong WF. The adrenal medulla and adrenal cortex. In Ganong WF (ed.) Review of Medical Physiology, 12th ed. Los Altos: Lange Medical Publications, 1985; 297.

68. Gibb DB. Suxamethonium – A review. Anaesth Intensive Care 1974; 2:9–26.

69. Giles CL. Tonometer tensions in the newborn. Arch Ophthalmol 1959; 61:517–519.

70. Goethals M, Missotten L. Intraocular pressure in children up to five years of age. J Pediatr Ophthalmol 1983; 20:49–51.

71. Goldmann H, Schmidt Th. Über Applanationstonometrie. Ophthalmologica 1957; 134:221–242.

72. Goldmann H. Abfluss des Kammerwassers beim Menschen. Ophthalmologica 1946; 111:146–152.

73. Goldmann H. Abflussdruck, Minutenvolumen und Widerstand der Kammerwasserströmung des Menschen. Docum Ophthalmol 1951; 5–6:278–356.

74. Goldmann H. Das Minutenvolumen der menschlichen Vorderkammer bei Normalen und bei Fällen von primärem Glaukom. Ophthalmologica 1950; 120:150–156.

75. Goldmann H. Un nouveau tonomètre à aplanation. Bull Soc Franç Ophtalmol 1955; 67:474–478.

76. Goldmann H, Schmidt. Ueber Tonometer. Ophthalmologica 1956; 131:335–341.

77. Goldmann H. Über Fluorescein in der menschlichen Vorderkammer. Das Kammerwasser-Minutenvolumen des Menschen. Ophthalmologica 1950; 119:65–95.

78. Gotoh I, Kitazawa Y. Intraocular pressure in newborn infants. Jpn J Ophthalmol 1968; 12:41–49.

79. Grant WM. Further studies on facility of flow through the trabecular meshwork. Arch Ophthalmol 1958; 60:523–533.

80. Green K, Pederson JE. Contribution of secretion and filtration to aqueous humor formation. Am J Physiol 1973; 222:1218–1226.

81. Grierson I, and Lee WR. Pressure-induced changes in the ultrastructure of the endothelium linig Schlemm's canal. Am J Ophthalmol 1975; 80:863–884.

82. Grierson I, Lee WR. Changes in the monkey outflow apparatus at graded levels of intraocular pressure: a quantitative analysis by light microscopy and scanning electron microscopy. Exp Eye Res 1974; 19:21–33.

83. Grierson I, Lee WR. The fine structure of the trabecular meshwork at graded levels of intraocular pressure. (1) Pressure effects within the near-physiological range (8–30 mmHg). Exp Eye Res 1975; 20:505–521.

84. Grierson I, Lee, WR, Abraham S. The appearance of the outflow apparatus of the eye after staining with ruthenium red. Acta Ophthalmol 1977; 55:827–836.

85. Grierson I, Robins E, Howes RC. Preliminary observations on human trabecular meshwork cells in vitro. Albrecht v Graefe's Arch Klin Exp Ophthalmol 1980; 212:173–186.

86. Grote P. Augeninnendruckmessungen bei Kleinkindern ohne Glaukom in Halothanmaskennarkose. Ophthalmologica 1975; 171:202–206.

87. Hara K, Lütjen-Drecoll E, Prestle H, Rohen JW. Structural differences between regions of ciliary body in primates. Invest Ophthalmol Vis Sci 1977; 16:912–924.

88. Harnisch JP. Elektronmikroskopische Darstellung sauer Mukopolysaccharide im Trabekelwerk. Klin Mbl Augenheilk 1976; 169:90–94.

89. Heinzen H. Effet de l'acétazoléamide (Diamox) sur le transfert du sodium radioactif (24Na) à travers la barrière hémato-aqueuse. Bull Soc Fr Ophthalmol 1955; 68:79–82.

90. Henderson Th. Significance of pressure equilibrum on the intraocular contents and its bearing on glaucoma and its treatment. Acta XVI Concil Ophthalmol 1951; 2:835–845.

91. Henriksson S, Holm O, Krakau CET. On the apparent size of structures in the anterior chamber. Acta Ophthalmol 1968; 46:278–283.

92. Hernandez MR, Weinstein BI, Wenk EJ, Gordon GG, Dunn MW, Southren AL. The effect of dexamethasone on the In vitro incorporation of precursors of extracellular matrix components in the outflow pathway region of the rabbit eye. Invest Ophthalmol Vis Sci 1983; 24:704–709.

93. Hernandez MR, Wenk EJ, Weinstein BI, Abumohor P, Podos SM, Dunn MW, Southren AL. Glucocorticoid target cells in human outflow pathway: autopsy and surgical specimens. Invest Ophthalmol Vis Sci 1983; 24:1612–1616.

94. Holm O, Krakau CET. A method of measuring pupillary aqueous flow. Acta Ophthalmol 1968; 46:558–563.

95. Holm O, Krakau CET. A photogrammetric method for estimation of the volume of superficial tumours and similar objects. Acta Univiversitatis Lundensis, Secto II, 1965; 31.

96. Holm O, Wiebert O. A photogrammetric method for estimation of the pupillary aqueous flow in the living human eye, II. Acta Ophthalmol 1968; 46:1230–1250.

97. Holm O. A photogrammetric method for estimation of the pupillary aqueous aqueous flow in the living human eye, I. Acta Ophthalmol 1968; 46:254–277.

98. Hörven I. Tonometry in newborn infants. Acta Ophthalmol 1961; 39:911–918.

99. Imbert A. Théorie des ophtalmotonomètres. Arch Ophtalmol (Paris) 1885; 5:358–363.

100. Inomata H, Bill A, Smelser GK. Aqueous humor pathways through the trabecular meshwork and into Schlemm's canal in the cynomolgus monkey (Macaca irus). An electron microscopic study. Am J Ophthalmol 1972; 73:760–789.

101. Johnstone M, Tanner D, Chau B, Kopecky K. Concentration-dependent morphologic effects of cytochalasin B in the aqueous outflow system. Invest Ophthalmol Vis Sci 1980; 19:835–841.

102. Jones TR, Reid TW. Trace Elements in the Eye. In Sears ML (ed.) Pharmacology of the Eye. Berlin: Springer-Verlag, 1984, pp. 678–679.

103. Kaufman PL, Bárány EH. Cytochalasin B reversibly increases outflow facility in the eye of the cynomolgus monkey. Invest Opthalmol Vis Sci 1977; 16:47–53.

104. Kaufman PL, Bárány EH. Recent observations concerning the effects of cholinergic drugs on outflow facility in monkeys. Exp Eye Res 1977; 25 (Suppl):415–418.

105. Kaufman PL, Erickson KA. Cytochalasin B and D does-outflow facility relationships in the cynomolgus monkey. Invest Ophthalmol Vis Sci 1982; 23:646–650.

106. Kaufman PL, Svedbergh B, Lütjen-Drecoll E. Medical trabeculocanalotomy in monkeys with cytochalasin B or EDTA. Ann Ophthalmol 1979; 11:795–796.

107. Kaye GI, Pappas GD. Studies on the ciliary epithelium and zonule. III. The fine stucture of the rabbit ciliary epithelium in relation to the localization of ATPase activity. J Microscopie 1965; 4:497–508.

108. Kielar RA, Teraslinna P, Kearney ST, Barker D. Effet of changes in PCO2 on intraocular tension. Invest Ophthalmol Vis Sci 1977; 16:534–537.

109. Kiss F. Der Blutkreislauf des Auges. Ophthalmologica 1943; 106:225–250.

110. Klyce SD, Palkama KA, Härkönen M, Marshall WS, Huhtaniitty S, Mann KP, Neufeld AH. Neural serotonin stimulates chloride transport in the rabbit corneal epithelium. Invest Ophthalmol Vis Sci 1982; 23:181–192.

111. Knepper PA, Farbman AI, Tesler AG. Aqueous outflow pathway glycosaminoglycans. Exp Eye Res 1981; 32:265–277.

112. Knepper PA, Farbman AI, Tesler AG. Exogenous hyaluronidases and degradation of hyaluronic acid in the rabbit eye. Invest Ophthalmol Vis Sci 1984; 25:286–293.

113. Kolker AE, Hetherington J. Becker-Shaffer's Diagnostic and therapy of the glaucomas, 5th ed. St. Louis: The C.V. Mosby Company, 1983; 59–60.

114. Korhonen E, Korhonen LK. Histochemical demonstration of carbonic anhydrase activity in the eyes of rat and mouse. Acta Ophthalmol 1965; 43:475–481.

115. Kornblueth W, Abrahamov A, Aladjemoff L, Magora F, Gombos G. Intraocular pressure in the newborn measured under general anesthesia. Arch Ophthalmol 1959; 61: 750–752.

116. Krakau CET. On the regulation of the intraocular pressure. The Bjerrum Memorial Lecture in the Danish Ophthalmological Society. Acta Ophthalmol 1969; 47:1069–1088.

117. Krupin T, Feitl M, Roshe R, Lee S, Becker B. Halothane anesthesia and aqueous humor dynamics in rabbit eyes. Invest Ophthalmol Vis Sci 1980; 19:518–521.

118. Laurent UBG. Hyaluronate in aqueous humor. Exp Eye Res 1981; 33:147–155.

119. Laurent UBG. Hyaluronate in human aqueous humor. Arch Ophthalmol 1983; 101: 129–130.

120. Leibowitz HM, Krueger DE, Maunder LR, Milton RC, Kini MM, Kahn HA, Nickerson RJ, Pool J, Colton TL, Ganley JP, Loewenstein JI, Dawber TR. The Framingham Eye Study Monograph. IV. Glaucoma. Surv Ophthalmol 1980; 4 (Suppl):335–400.

121. Lewallen WM, Hicks BL. The use of succinylcholine in ocular surgery. Am J Ophthalmol 1960; 49:773–780.

122. Leydhecker W, Réhak S, Mathyl J. Untersuchungen zur Homöostasis: Der Einfluss experimenteller Druckänderungen auf die Kammerwasserproduktion des lebenden Kaninchenauges. Klin Mbl Augenheilk 1971; 159:427–430.

123. Leys M, van Rij G, de Heer LJ. The influence of oxybuprocaine (Novesine) on the intraocular pressure. Doc Ophthalmol 1986; 61:295–301.

124. Lindner K. Zur Untersuchung des Flüssigkeitswechels in Auge. Dtsch Ophthalmol 1920; 42:33–49.

125. Loewen U, Handrup B, Redeker A. Results of a glaucoma mass sceening program. Klin Mbl Augenheilk 1976; 169:754–766.

126. Luly P, Barnabei O, Tria E. Hormonal control in vitro of plasma membrane-bound Na^+K^+-ATPase of rat liver. Biochim Biophys Acta 1972; 282:447–452.

127. Lütjen-Drecoll E, Lönnerholm G, Eichhorn M. Carbonic anhydrase distribution in the human and monkey eye by light and electron microscopy. Graefe's Arch Clin Exp Ophthalmol 1983; 220:285–291.

128. Lütjen-Drecoll E, Lönnerholm G, Ober M. Carbonic anhydrase activity in the monkey anterior ocular segment. Invest Ophthalmol Vis Sci 1978; 17 (Suppl):162.

129. Maddox TS, Kielar RA. Comparison of the influence of ketamine and halothane anesthesia on intraocular tensions of on glaucomatous children. J Pediatr Ophthalmol 1974; 11:90–93.

130. Maklakoff. L'ophtalmotonométrie. Arch Ophtalmol (Paris) 1885; 5:159–165.

131. Malina HZ, Martin XD. Hydroxyindole-O-methyltransferase activity in human iris/ciliary body. Abstract. Eur J Neurosc 1991; 4 (Suppl):228.

132. Mao LK, Stewart WC, Shields MB. Correlation between intraocular pressure control and progessive glaucomatous damage in primary open-angle glaucoma. Am J Ophthalmol 1991; 111:51–55.

133. Martin XD. Letter to the Editor. Invest Ophthalmol Vis Sci 1992; 33:3480.

134. Martin XD, Brennan MC, Lichter PR. Serotonin in human aqueous humor. Ophthalmology 1988; 95:1221–1226.

135. Martin XD, Malina HZ, Brennan MC, Hendrickson PH, Lichter PR. The ciliary body – The third organ found to synthesize indoleamines in human. Euro J ophthalmol 1992; 2:67–72.

136. Martin XD. Normal intraocular pressure in man. Ophthalmologica 1992; 205:57–63.

137. Meyer K, Palmer JW. On the nature of the ocular fluids. Am J Ophthalmol 1936; 19:859–865.

138. Mizokami K. Demonstration of masked acidic glycosamino-glycans in the normal human trabecular meshwork. Jpn J Ophthalmol 1977; 21:57–71.

139. Moreno RJ, Kloess P, Carlson DW. Effect of succinylcholine on the intraocular contents of open globes. Ophthalmology 1991; 98:636–638.

140. Morsman CD. Letter to the editor. Ophthalmology 1991; 98:1607–1608.

141. Moseley H, Grierson I, Lee WR. Mathematical modelling of aqueous humour outflow from the eye through the pores in the lining endothelium of Schlemm's canal. Clin Phys Physiol Meas 1983; 4:47–63.

142. Moses RA. The Goldmann applanation tonometer. Am J Ophthalmol 1958; 46:865–869.

143. Perkins ES. Glaucoma screening from a public health clinic. Br Med J 1965; 1:417–419.

144. Petounis AD, Chondreli S, Vadaluka-Sekioti A. Effect of hypercapnea and hyperventilation on human intraocular pressure during general anesthesia following acetazolamide administration. Br J Ophthalmol 1980; 64:422–425.

145. Polanski JR, Gospodarowicz D, Weinreb RN, Alvarado JJ. Human trabecular meshwork cell culture and glycosamino-glycan synthesis. Invest Ophthalmol Vis Sci 1978; 17 (Suppl):207.

146. Radtke ND, Cohan BE. Intraocular pressure measurement in the newborn. Am J Ophthalmol 1974; 78:501–504.

147. Radtke N, Waldmann J. The influence of enflurane anesthesia on intraocular pressure in youths. Anesth Analg 1975; 54:212–215.

148. Reiss GR, Lee DA, Topper JE, and Brubaker RF. Aqueous humor flow during sleep. Invest. Ophthalmol Vis Sci 1984; 25:776–778.

149. Richardson T. distribution of glycosaminoglycans in the aqueous outflow system of the cat. Invest Ophthalmol Vis Sci 1982; 22:319–329.

150. Riley MV. The sodium-potassium-stimulated adenosine triphosphate of rabbit ciliary epithelium. Exp Eye Res 1964; 3:76–84.

151. Ruprecht KW, Wulle KG, Christl HL. Applanation tonometry within medical diagnostic "check-up" programs. Klin Mbl Augenheilk 1978; 172:332–341.

152. Sampaolesi R. La pression oculaire et le sinus camérulaire chez l'enfant normal et dans le glaucome congénital au-dessus de l'âge de cinq ans. Doc Ophthalmol 1969; 26:497–515.

153. Samuel JR, Beaugié A. Effect of carbon dioxyde on the intraocular pressure in man during general anaesthesia. Br J Ophthalmol 1974; 58:62–67.

154. Schachtschabel B, Bigalke B, Rohen JW. Production of glycosaminoglycans by cell cultures of the trabecular meshwork of the primate eye. Exp Eye Res 1977; 24:71–80.

155. Schiøtz Hj. Ein neuer Tonometer. – Tonometrie. Arch Augenheilk 1905; 52:401–424.

156. Schreck E. Zur intravitalen Modelldarstellung des Flüssigkeitswechsels im Menschenauge. Ber Dtsch Ophthal Ges 1949; 55:174–178.

157. Schreuder M, Linssen GH. Intraocular pressure and anesthesia. Direct measurement by needling the anterior chamber in the monkey. Anesthesia 1972; 27:165–170.

158. Seiler T, Wollensak J. The resistance of the trabecular meshwork to aqueous humor outflow. Graefe's Arch Clin Exp Ophthalmol 1985; 223:88–91.

159. Self WG, Ellis PP. The effect of general anesthetic agents on intraocular pressure. Surv Ophthalmol 1977; 21:494–500.

160. Shields MB. Textbook of Glaucoma, 2nd ed. Baltimore: Williams & Wilkins, 1987; 45–46.

161. Shiose Y, Sears ML. Fine structural localization of nucleoside phosphatase activity in the ciliary epithelium of albino rabbits. Invest Ophthalmol 1966; 5:152–165.

162. Southren AL, Gordon GG, L'Hommedieu D, Ravikumar S, Dunn MW, Weinstein BI. 5-β-dihydroxy-cortisol: possible mediator of the ocular hypertension in glaucoma. Invest Ophthalmol Vis Sci 1985; 26:393–395.

163. Southren AL, Gordon GG, Munnangi PR, Vittek J, Schwarz J, Monder C, Dunn MW, Weinstein BI. Altered cortisol metabolism in cells cultured from trabecular meshwork specimens obtained from patients with primary open-angle glaucoma. Invest Ophthalmol Vis Sci 1983; 24:1413–1417.

164. Sugar HS. Experimental trabeculectomy in glaucoma. Am J Ophthalmol 1961; 51:623–627.

165. Svedbergh B, Lütjen-Drecoll E, Ober M, Kaufman PL. Cytochalasin B-induced structural changes in the anterior ocular segment of the cynomolgus monkey. Invest Ophthalmol Vis Sci 1978; 17:718–734.

166. Tammisto T, Hämäläinen L, Tarkkanen L. Halothane and methoxyflurane in ophthalmic anesthesia. Acta Anaesthesiol Scand 1965; 9:173–177.

167. Thomas RC. Membrane current and intracellular sodium changes in a snail neurone during extrusion of injected sodium. J Physiol (London) 1969; 201:495–514.

168. Topper JE, Brubaker RF. Effects of timolol, epinephrine, and acetazolamide on aqueous flow during sleep. Invest Ophthalmol Vis Sci 1985; 26:1315–1319.

169. Tormay A, Ortega M, Mittag T. Calcium/calmodulin-activated adenylate cyclase in rabbit ciliary process membranes. Invest Ophthalmol Vis Sci 1987; 28 (Suppl):285.

170. Tripathi RC, Tripathi BJ. Sialic acid moieties in the human trabecular meshwork. Invest Ophthalmol Vis Sci 1987; 28 (Suppl):284.

171. Tripathi RC. Mechanism of aqueous outflow across the trabecular wall of Schlemm's canal. Exp Eye Res 1971; 11:116–121.

172. Tripathi RC. Pressure-dependency of aqueous outflow. Am J Ophthalmol 1973; 76: 402–403.

173. Tripathi RC. The aqueous outflow in normal and glaucomatous eyes. Br J Ophthalmol 1972; 56:157–174.

174. Tripathi RC. The functional morphology of the outflow systems of ocular and cerebrospinal fluids. Exp Eye Res 1977; 25 (Suppl):65–116.

175. Tripathi RC. Ultrastructure of the exit pathway of aqueous in lower mammals: a preliminary report on the "angular aqueous plexus." Exp Eye Res 1971; 12:311–314.

176. Tripathi RC. Ultrastucture of Schlemm's canal in relation to aqueous outflow. Exp Eye Res 1968; 7:335–341.

177. Troncoso U, Castroviejo R. Microanatomy of the eye with slit lamp microscope: I. Comparative anatomy of the angle of the anterior chamber in living and sectioned eyes of mammalia. Am J Ophthalmol 1936; 19:371–384.

178. Troncoso U, Castroviejo R. Microanatomy of the eye with slit lamp microscope: II. Comparative anatomy of the angle of the anterior chamber in living and sectioned eyes of mammalia. Am J Ophthalmol 1936; 19:481–492.

179. Troncoso U, Castroviejo R. Microanatomy of the eye with slit lamp microscope: III. Comparative anatomy of the angle of the anterior chamber in living and sectioned eyes of mammalia. Am J Ophthalmol 1936; 19:583–592.

180. Troncoso U. La filtration dans l'oeil vivant et la nature véritable du canal de Schlemm. Ann Ocul 1909; 142:237–265.

181. Troncoso U. Recherches expérimentales sur la filtration des liquides salins et albumineux à travers la chambre antérieure et son rôle dans la genèse du glaucome. Ann Ocul 1905; 133:5–31.

182. Troncoso U. The physiologic nature of the Schlemm canal. Am J Ophthalmol 1921; 4:321–326.

183. Trope GE, Rumley AG. Catecholamines in human aqueous humor. Invest Ophthalmol Vis Sci 1985; 26:399–401.

184. Warner DM, Chu EB. The role of ionic calcium in the resistance to aqueous outflow in the cat. Can J Ophthalmol 1967; 2:226–232.

185. Weekers R, Demarcelle Y. Mesure du débit de l'humeur aqueuse. Etude de 180 cas. Ophthalmologica 1954; 127:373–385.

186. Weekers R. Considérations sur l'écoulement de l'humeur aqueuse. Ann Ocul 1951; 184:696–706.

187. Weinreb RN, Bloom E, Baxter JD, Alvarado J, Lan N, O'Donnell J, Polansky JR. Detection of glucocorticoid receptors in cultured human trabecular cells. Invest Ophthalmol Vis Sci 1981; 21:403–407.

188. Weinstein BI, Gordon GG, Southren AL. Potentiation of glucocorticoid activity by 5-β-dihydrocortisol: its role in glaucoma. Science 1983; 222:172–173.

189. Weinstein BI, Munnangi P, Gordon GG, Southren AL. Defects in cortisol-metabolizing enzymes in primary open-angle glaucoma. Invest Ophthalmol Vis Sci 1985; 26: 890–893.

190. Wessells NK, Spooner BS, Ash JF, Bradley MO, Luduena MA, Taylor EL, Wrenn JT, Yamada KM. Microfilaments in cellular and developmental processes. Contractile microfilament machinery of many cell types is reversibly inhibited by cytochalasin B. Science 1971; 171:135–143.

191. Whitacre MM, Emig M, Hassanein K. The effect of Perkins, Tono-Pen, and Schiøtz Tonometry on intraocular pressure. Am J Ophthalmol 1991; 111:59–64.

192. Wistrand PJ, Garg LC. Evidence of a high-activity C type of carbonic anhydrase in human ciliary processes. Invest Ophthalmol Vis Sci 1979; 18:802–806.

193. Wistrand PJ. Carbonic anhydrase in the anterior uvea of the rabbit. Acta Physiol Scand 1951; 24:144–148.
194. Worthen DM, Cleveland PH. Fibronectin production by cultured human trabecular meshwork cells. Invest Ophthalmol Vis Sci 1982; 23:265–269.
195. Yoshimura K. Activation of NaK activated ATPase in rat brain by catecholamine. J Biochem 1973; 74:389–391.
196. Zimmerman LE. Demonstration of hyaluronidase-sensitive acid mucopolysaccharide. Am J Ophthalmol 1957; 44:1–4.
197. Zumbrun FA, Weinberg RN, Alvarado JA, Polanski JR. Endogenous hyaluronidase and degradation of hyaluronic acid by human trabecular cells. Invest Ophthalmol Vis Sci 1981; 20 (Suppl):23.

CHAPTER 4
THE PHARMACOLOGY OF AQUEOUS HUMOR DYNAMICS

4.1 Introduction

The major contribution of Duke-Elder [102, 104, 105, 106, 107] on aqueous humor makes it imperative to begin this chapter by recalling his text on "The formation of the aqueous humor" [101]:

> "Since the basis of this active process [the formation of the aqueous humour] is a complex series of biochemical reactions it is reasonable to hope that this could be interrupted in a number of places by suitable enzymatic inhibitors, so that the therapeutic agents, such as acetazoleamide [sic], already at our disposal may be increased in number and perhaps in effectiveness in the future."

What was true for acetazolamide in 1968 is true today for β-blockers. Indeed, as shown below, it is possible that the main action of β-blockers could be the reduction of serotonin stimulation of Na^+K^+-ATPase in the nonpigmented ciliary epithelium [231].

If an understanding of the biochemical cascades is prerequisite to rational influence on aqueous humor formation, it is obvious that a perfect understanding of this mechanism of secretion is the *sine qua non* condition for progress in its pharmacological control and modulation. Although the specific action for a drug in a certain level is probably often possible, it is nevertheless not enough, since other tissues or organs are susceptible to using the same mechanism, thus explaining some side effects. Pharmacology must therefore develop not only specific drugs, but also a new *concept of specificity* of the drug to a certain site, with minimum effect on the others.

4.2 Drugs Acting on the Inflow System

4.2.1 Carboanhydrase Inhibitors

Since its discovery in the erythrocytes of the ox by Meldrum and Roughton [259, 260], the enzyme carbonic anhydrase has been found in a variety of organs, particularly in the ciliary body of the eye by Wistrand [390].

Both Friedenwald's hypothesis [131] for the active transport of electrolytes into the eye by the ciliary body as well as the determination of a high concentration of bicarbonate in the posterior chamber by Kinsey [186] led Becker [23] and Grant et al. [148] to test the effects of acetazolamide, a carbonic anhydrase inhibitor, on the intraocular pressure in humans. It was only in 1959 that Kinsey and Reddy [187] demonstrated that acetazolamide inhibits bicarbonate formation, a finding confirmed by Maren in 1976 [229], who postulated that this phenomenon was the pharmacological basis for a decrease in aqueous humor production.

Acetazolamide is the most commonly used carboanhydrase inhibitor of aqueous humor production, although other drugs, in particular methazolamide, but also dichlophenamide and ethoxzolamide, have been investigated.

Mechanism of Action[1]

Carbonic anhydrase inhibition by acetazolamide produces cascade reactions that are not yet completely understood. The *primum movens* of the mechanism of action is probably the inhibition of the enzyme, since acetazolamide fails to decrease pressure in patients with carbonic anhydrase II (previously referred to as C) deficiency [199].

Inhibition of the transformation of $CO_2 + H_2O$ in $H + HCO_3$ produces a blockage of the H – Na pump. Since no H is present to be exchanged against Na, there is a decrease of sodium entry into the cell and, consequently, a decrease of the secretion of Na in the posterior chamber via intercellular channels. These modifications in intracellular ion composition can reduce the activity of the Na^+K^+-ATPase enzyme and, thus, of the sodium-potassium pump by two mechanisms: first, by decreasing available sodium and second by lowering the pH into the cell, inducing a metabolic acidosis [75, 112]. Therefore, local pH changes seem able to induce a certain Na^+K^+-ATPase inhibition as well as a decrease of aqueous humor production.

1 Carbonic anhydrase enzyme physiology was discussed in Chapter 3 on p. 18.

Quantitatively, carbonic anhydrase inhibitors decrease the aqueous flow in the normal human eye by 20–27% [86] during the day and by 2% during the night [361].

Although not directly correlated with aqueous humor dynamics, acetazolamide does increase the urinary excretion of bicarbonate and fixed cations, mostly sodium, which involves a decrease in the concentration of bicarbonate in the extracellular fluid and the development of metabolic acidosis [383]. On the other hand and as a consequence of this acidosis [343], acetazolamide is known to be a cerebral vasodilator in both animals and humans [266] as well as a choroidal [388] and a retinal [365] vasodilator in monkeys. This increased blood flow after acetazolamide could explain the partial reversibility in the glaucomatous visual-field defects observed by Flammer and Drance [126] and before them by Paterson [304] and Heilmann [153]. However, the diuretic effect [305] and the ocular blood flow changes do not seem to be involved in the pressure decrease induced by acetazolamide [36].

As already shown by Davenport [88] in red cells and by Maren [228] in ocular tissues, more than 99% of the carbonic anhydrase had to be inhibited before a pharmacological effect was observed. This could explain why about 40 years were necessary since the introduction of acetazolamide as an ocular hypotensive drugs in 1954 [23, 145] until dorzolamide hydrochloride 2%, a topical preparation, was synthesized and found to be equipotent with the carboanhydrase inhibitors administered systemically [120, 148, 189].

4.2.2 Adrenergic Inhibitors

4.2.2.1 β_1 *and* β_2*-Blockers*

A. β-Blockers Without Intrinsic Sympathomimetic Activity (without ISA)

a. L-Timolol Maleate (L-{-}-1-{t-Butylamino}-3-{(4-morpholino-1, 2, 5-Thiadiazol-3- yl)oxy}-2-Propanol)

"Great interest has been shown in many compounds which have been employed for the therapy of systemic hypertension" – thus, Irving H. Leopold began his chapter on the antihypertensive ocular drugs in the first publication of *Survey of Ophthalmology* in 1956 [210]. Among these compounds is isoproterenol, a powerful nonselective β-agonist applied topically, producing a hypotensive ocular effect observed the previous year by Weekers [381]. So began this "marathon," which continued with the commercialization of the first ocular β-blocker in 1978. Thirty-one years after his 1956 publication, Irving H. Leopold [211] wrote:

"In summary, the mechanism of action of β-blocking agents in lowering intraocular pressure has not been fully established. It has been shown that β-blockers substantially reduce aqueous humor formation, and it has been suggested that they may do this independent of their interaction with β-adrenergic receptors of the ciliary processes."

Recently, Liu and Chiou [218] showed that the dextro-isomer of timolol, with its low affinity for β-receptors, may be as effective in decreasing aqueous flow as is the levo-isomer of timolol. This in turn may support the idea of some other mechanism being responsible for the decrease in intraocular pressure [211].

If one supposes that the blockage of β-receptors is a good means for lowering the intraocular pressure, we may consider three possible mechanisms of action: (1) decrease of aqueous secretion (inflow), (2) increase the evacuation (outflow), or (3) both. The inflow is located in the ciliary body, and its β-receptors are mainly of the β_2 adrenergic subtype. The outflow occurs through the trabecular meshwork, and its β-receptors are also of the β_2 adrenergic subtype.

Best-known among the β-adrenergic blocking agents is timolol maleate, a β_1 and β_2 adrenergic antagonist.

Tonographic [346, 400] and fluorophotometric studies in cats [216], monkeys [263], and humans [69, 393] all indicate that timolol lowers the intraocular pressure by reducing aqueous humor production. "Logically" speaking, its effect of lowering ocular pressure has been attributed to the blockage of adrenergic β-receptors. However, many points support the hypothesis that this effect is not solely a consequence of a blockage of the ocular β-receptors.

(1) Specificity and Stereo-Specificity of β-Blockers

It is well known that the L-enantiomers of β-adrenergic antagonists are more active than the D-isomers [19], [316]. Moreover, the L-enantiomer of timolol, one of the most efficient β-blockers, is bound stereospecifically and nonspecifically to the β-receptors, whereas the d-isomer has low affinity for β-receptors [360]. While this is true for the cardiac muscle, according to Nathanson [283] it is not the case for the ciliary process in rabbit and in humans, where, with the exception of metoprolol, the R- or D-enantiomers of timolol, betaxolol, butylbetaxolol, bunitrolol, and didesmethyl-ICI-118,551 demonstrate a substantially higher absolute affinity for β_2-receptors. This could explain why D-timolol is as effective in decreasing aqueous flow as the L-isomer of timolol [218, 340].

Many β-blockers, including nonselective ones such as timolol, propanolol, sotolol, pindolol, bupranolol, and carteolol [47, 49, 69, 176, 287, 329], β_1-selective antagonists such as atenolol, metoprolol, [57, 111, 367, 386], and betaxolol [27], and β_2-selective antagonist H 35/25 [220] reduce intraocular pressure.

However, the β-receptors of the ciliary processes are predominantly β_2-receptors [55, 281, 282]. One explanation could be that β-blockers such as betaxolol also have a weak action on β_2-receptors, and that very small concentrations are able to block β_1- and β_2-receptors. Indeed, according to Nathanson [284] and his kinetic studies [283], betaxolol is not β_1-selective. It is, in fact, relatively nonselective (heat/ciliary process ratio of 1:1 for S- or L-betaxolol, compared with 1.2 for S-timolol). This explanation could be correct, since even the lowest concentrations of timolol, for example, can block *all* β_1- and β_2-receptors.

(2) Intraocular Pressure Effects after Unilateral Instillation

Timolol passes into the plasma after instillation [303, 331, 372] and into the contralateral ciliary body after unilateral instillation [368], which explains the systemic side effects. In the rabbit, the blood plasma concentration of timolol [331, 372] and the concentration of timolol in the contralateral ciliary body after unilateral instillation [368] were much higher than the dissociation constant and the inhibition constant for timolol in the iris-ciliary body [21, 291]. In humans, blood plasma concentration of timolol [303] is sufficient for this blockage to occur [282].

These data allow the assumption that, since timolol concentrations were higher or comparable to those necessary to block the β-receptors, in the treated eye as well as in the untreated eye, intraocular pressure should decrease equally in both eyes. This presumes that the decrease in intraocular pressure is the consequence of the β-blockage.

In order to verify whether a very low concentration of timolol that can block all β_1- and β_2-receptors was also able to lower the intraocular pressure, Martin and Rabineau [246] did the following study: Bilateral intraocular pressure curves were established in 14 normal, young subjects, four women and ten men between 23 and 39 years of age (average 29.9 years ± 4.3 SD) without current or previous ocular disease. The intraocular pressure of each eye in all subjects was measured at precisely 8:00 and 11:00 a.m. and 2:00 and 5:00 p.m. with a calibrated Goldmann applanation tonometer (Model T 900 Haag-Streit, Berne, Switzerland) preceding and 1 week after beginning timolol 0.5% instillation twice daily in one eye (at 7:00 a.m. and 8:00 p.m.). All subjects experienced a subsequent intraocular pressure decrease in the treated eye, but no subjects had a statistically significant intraocular pressure decrease in the contralateral eye. The mean intraocular pressure reduction of 26% ($2p < 0.00015$) in the treated eye was statistically highly significant (Fig. 6 A), and only 3% ($2p < 0.33$) in the contralateral eye was statistically not significant (Fig. 6 B). These results suggest that timolol does not normally lower intraocular pressure in the contralateral eye after unilateral instillation in normal subjects. Our results were recently confirmed by other authors, who found no statistically sig-

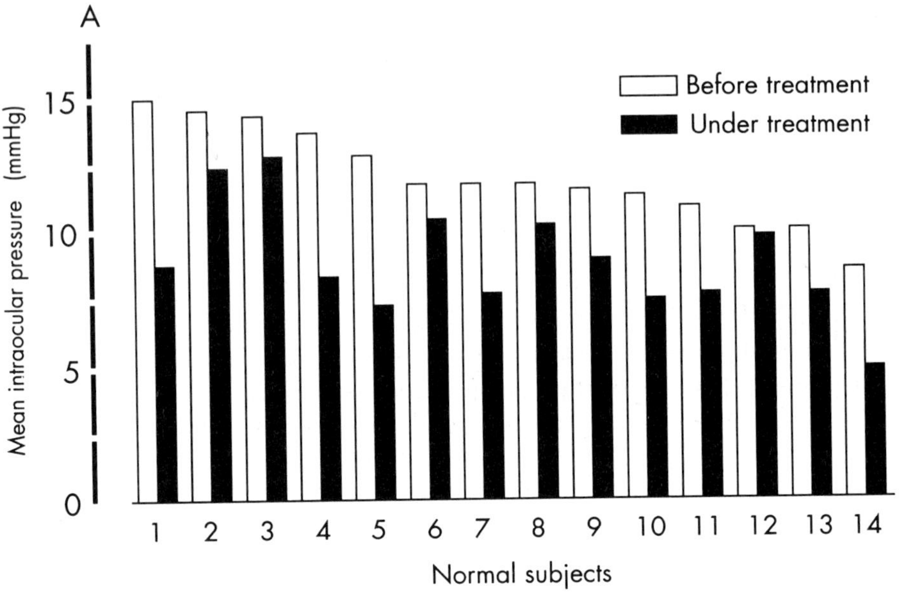

A. Mean intraocular pressure of timolol-treated eyes in 14 normal subjects before treatment (white) and under treatment (solid black).

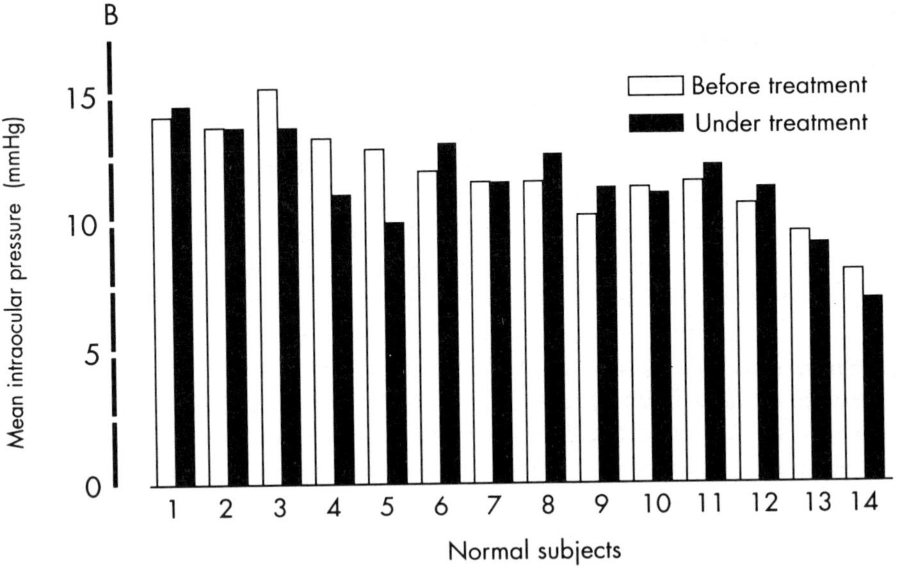

B. Mean intraocular pressure of contralateral untreated eyes in 14 normal subjects before treatment (white) and under treatment of partner eyes (solid black).

Figure 6. Intraocular pressure effects after unilateral instillation of timolol.

nificant decrease in contralateral eyes 2 hours after a single dose of 0.25% timolol [273]. The fact that intraocular pressure did not decrease symmetrically after unilateral instillation argues against β-blockage being only a mechanism of action of the hypotensive effect.

The fact that timolol is generally considered to lower intraocular pressure in both eyes after unilateral instillation is based mainly on three frequently cited studies. The first is the study in the rabbit by Vareilles et al. [372], in which it is clearly mentioned that both eyes had received timolol instillation. The second is Zimmerman and Kaufman's [402] study of glaucoma patients. The latter authors did not discuss the observed intraocular pressure decrease in the untreated eye – and that for good reason, since this decrease was not statistically significantly different from that observed in the placebo group. In a previous publication [401], however, these authors had noted an intraocular pressure decrease in the contralateral eye. The third study is by Radius et al. [315] in the rabbit, in which a significant decrease in IOP was measured in the contralateral eye after unilateral instillation. These results, however, contradict those of Vareilles et al. [372] and Bartels et al. [21], who had measured only insignificant effects on intraocular pressure after bilateral instillation in the rabbit. In the cat, Colasanti and Trotter [73] found no significant pressure reduction in the contralateral eyes.

However, in humans a decrease in intraocular pressure in the untreated eye has been reported in normal subjects [286, 347] and in glaucoma patients [286, 347, 401]. This decrease was usually smaller than that found in treated eyes, but statistically significant in some glaucoma patients nonetheless [347, 401]. Moreover, the difference between the treated and untreated eyes was also significant [401]. These last two findings are particularly important, as they allow us to suggest two different mechanisms of action for timolol depending on β-blockage, one local and one systemic. The local action could be the result of the vasoconstriction of ciliary vessels [117, 289, 320], and the systemic effect the result of the lowering of systemic blood pressure [262, 130]. The latter effect, the amplitude of which was lower, was observed only in patients with ocular hypertension and glaucoma, since it is known that the higher the initial intraocular pressure, the greater the hypotensive action of topical agents [195].

However, the results of Martin and Rabineau [246] show that, in normal subjects, any decrease in the intraocular pressure in the contralateral eye is not statistically significant; these results support the observations of Spinelli et al. [347]. Such findings suggest that the lowering of the intraocular pressure in treated eyes induced by β-blockers is, at least in some part, induced by local and systemic β-blockage and, for the greater part, the consequence of local action, though the mechanism remains unclear.

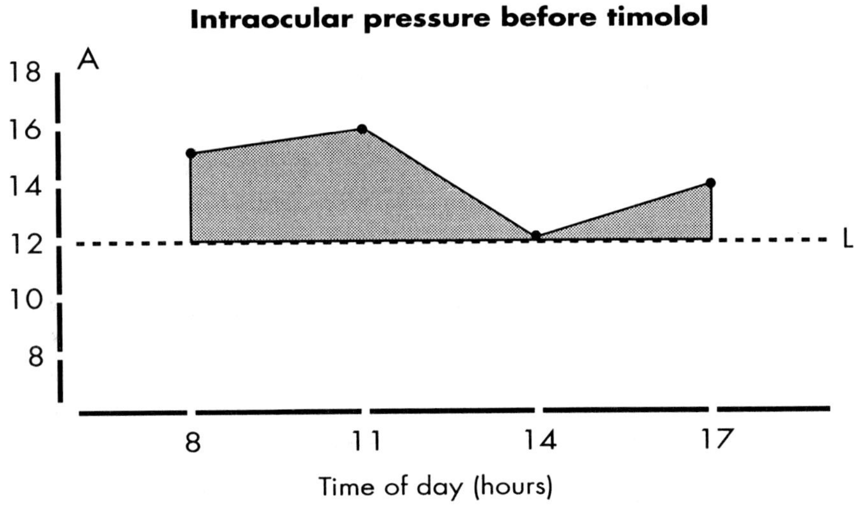

A. Intraocular pressure measurements before timolol: the area under the curve is 19.7 surface units (mmHg × hour).

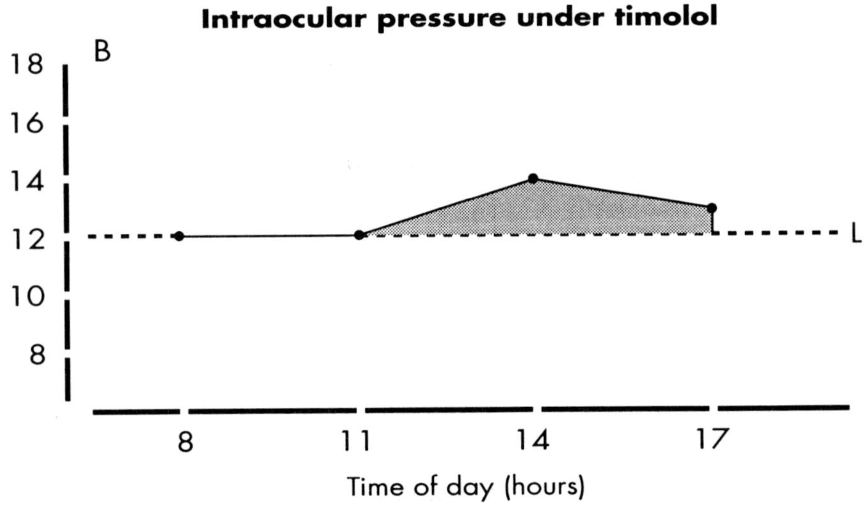

B. Intraocular pressure measurements under timolol: the area under the curve is only 7.5 surface units. The area reduction in this case is 12 surface units, i.e., 61.5%. These curves are those from the 20th subject on the histogram in Figure 8.

Figure 7. Method of measurement of the amplitude of diurnal variations of intraocular pressure.
The area under the curve from each eye before and under timolol therapy was calculated relative to the baseline (L), corresponding to the lowest intraocular pressure measured. The shaded area is that which was measured.

(3) Timolol Decreases the Amplitude of Diurnal Variations of Intraocular Pressure

In a study comparing the effect of pilocarpine and timolol on the intraocular pressure in eight open-angle glaucoma patients, Hass and Drance [151] observed a flattening effect in the diurnal curves of seven eyes under timolol which had not occurred under pilocarpine. The statistically undersized collective and the absence of correlation with pressure curves before treatment prevented them from interpreting those results. However, the proceeding clinical impression is interesting if one considers the mechanisms of action of pilocarpine and timolol.

Since diurnal variations of intraocular pressure are probably related to indoleamines, catecholamines, prostaglandines, and the sensory nervous system; and because timolol is able to block β_1, β_2, and to reduce dopamine concentration in iris root-ciliary body [376] as well as to act like an antagonist of serotonin [190], Martin et al. [247] evaluated the effect of timolol on diurnal variations in intraocular pressure.

A total of 88 intraocular pressure curves were established in 22 normal young volunteers. Intraocular pressure was measured in both eyes before and 1 week after the beginning of monolateral treatment with timolol 0.5% twice daily. The method of measurement is described in Figure 7 A and 7 B.

The results showed a decrease in amplitude of diurnal variations of 24% ($p = 0.07$ in paired t-test) in timolol-treated eyes (Fig. 8 A.) and no significant change in the contralateral eyes (Fig. 8 B.). The difference between both eyes was statistically significant in paired t-test ($p = 0.01$).

This anticircadian effect of timolol is very interesting and must be considered in the light of the observations of Topper and Brubacker [361], who found that timolol had no action on aqueous flow during sleep.

(4) Effects of Timolol on Visual-Field Parameters

In a single-blind, randomized study on visual fields of 12 normal young subjects (average 30.6 ± 4.2 years) measured three times at weekly intervals, Martin et al. [245] analyzed the fluctuations in visual field parameters using program G1 of the Octopus 500 Automated Perimeter. The visual fields were measured 1 week and 1 day before therapy and a third time 1 week after beginning unilateral instillation of one drop of timolol 0.5% twice daily. The mean sensitivity, the corrected loss variance, the short-term fluctuations, and the reliability factor were calculated for both eyes. The paired t-test was used. In statistical analysis, a p-value < 0.05 indicated significance and a p-value between 0.1 and 0.05 indicated trend.

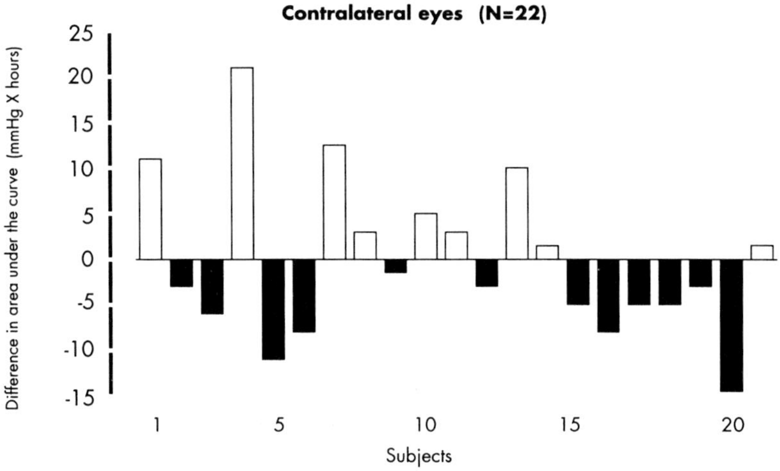

A. Difference in area under the curve (i. e., mmHg plotted against time) between the pressure curves of further (further = the eye which will be treated) treated eyes and the same eyes under timolol. Seventeen of 22 subjects present a decrease of the area under the curve, that is to say, a decrease of the intraocular pressure diurnal changes. The mean decrease was 24.2% ($p = 0.07$).

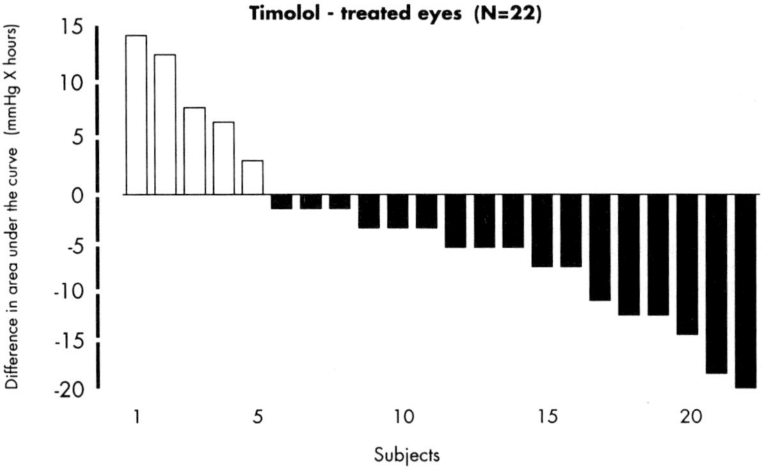

B. Difference in area under the curve between the pressure curves before and under timolol for contralateral untreated eyes. The 22 subjects were aleatorily distributed. The mean decrease of the diurnal amplitude variations of the intraocular pressure was 1.4% ($p = 0.9$).

Figure 8. Amplitude difference between the diurnal variations before and under timolol 0.5%. These two histograms represent the amplitude changes of intraocular pressure diurnal variations of twenty-two subjects classed by decreasing order of change amplitude of the treated eye.

Table 4. Measurements of Visual Fields (dB) (mean ± SD).

One week before treatment (Condition 1)
One day before treatment (Condition 2)
One week after beginning of treatment (Condition 3)

Eyes	Mean Sensitivity (dB)	Corrected loss variance (dB)	Short-term fluctuations (dB)	Reliability factor
Condition 1				
Future timolol-treated eyes (n = 11)	28.95 ± 0.71	1.55 ± 0.86	1.27 ± 0.23	2.05 ± 2.06
Future fellow eyes (n = 11)	29.11 ± 0.64	1.89 ± 1.17	1.25 ± 0.20	2.20 ± 3.65
Condition 2				
Future timolol-treated eyes (n = 11)	28.89 ± 0.55	2.16 ± 1.99	1.41 ± 0.23	3.00 ± 3.70
Future fellow eyes (n = 11)	28.88 ± 0.54	2.58 ± 3.46	1.37 ± 0.29	2.41 ± 3.28
Condition 3				
Timolol treated-eyes (n = 11)	28.92 ± 0.79	1.96 ± 2.07	1.22 ± 0.16	1.84 ± 1.82
Contralateral eyes (n = 11)	28.67 ± 0.57	1.96 ± 1.72	1.30 ± 0.09	0.84 ± 1.52

Table 5. Statistical Analysis of Mean Sensitivity.

	D	SD	T	*p*
Timolol-treated eyes (n = 11)				
Visual field 1 against 3	–0.03	0.90	–0.10	not significant
Visual field 2 against 3	+0.04	0.65	0.18	not significant
Contralateral eyes (n = 11)				
Visual field 1 against 3 significant	–0.44	0.51	–2.82	< 0.01
Visual field 2 against 3	–0.21	0.54	–1.29	$0.1 < p < 0.25$
Timolol-treated against contralateral (n = 22)				
Visual field 1 against 3 trend	0.41	0.78	1.74	$0.05 < p < 0.1$
Visual field 2 against 3	0.25	0.68	1.24	$0.1 < p < 0.25$

The paired t-test was used. In statistical analysis, a *p*-value ≤ 0.05 indicates significance and a *p*-value between 0.1 and 0.05 indicates trend. D = Difference; SD = Standard Deviation.

Table 4 gives the mean value of all measurements of visual field parameters and Table 5 the statistical analysis of mean sensitivity.

Whereas after 1 week of instillation no statistically significant effect was found in the treated eyes (Fig. 9 A), the contralateral, untreated eyes showed

Table 6. Mean arterial blood pressure.

A. Mean blood pressure before and under timolol 0.5% twice a day in one eye for one week

Subjects (n = 12)		Mean arterial blood pressure (mmHg)			
		Before timolol		Under timolol	
	Age	Right arm	Left arm	Right arm	Left arm
Mean	30.6	114.6/76.2	110.8/72.9	107.5/72.1	106.2/70.4
SD	± 4.25	±11.2/±11.5	±10.6/±10.3	±10.1/±10.1	±9.1/±8.4

B. Mean blood pressure decrease under timolol 0.5% twice daily in one eye for one week

Subjects (n = 12)	Mean blood pressure decrease (mmHg)			
	Right arm		Left arm	
	Systolic	Diastolic	Systolic	Diastolic
mmHg	−6.67 ± 8.07	−4.17 ±12.76	−4.58 ± 6.20	−2.5 ± 10.34
%	−5.8%	−5.4%	−4.1%	−3.4%
T	−2.86	−1.13	−2.56	−0.84
$p <$	0.01	–	0.025	–

a statistically significant decrease of mean sensitivity between the first visual fields and the third ones ($p < 0.01$) (Fig. 9 B and 10).

Arterial blood pressure was measured in both arms 1 day before treatment began and then after 1 week of instillation. The results are shown in Table 6. Systolic arterial blood pressure decreased 5%, and diastolic pressure decreased 4.4%. These results were statistically significant ($p < 0.01$ for right arms and 0.025 for left arms in paired t-test) for the systolic decrease, but not so for the diastolic reduction (Tab. 6).

The reduction of mean sensitivity in the untreated contralateral eyes may be due to systemic side effects (lowering of the blood pressure and slowing of cardiac frequency) not compensated for by local lowering of intraocular pressure in normal subjects.

Confirmation of these results might mean that the local and systemic β-blockage effects on the untreated eyes in the absence of significant lowering in the untreated eye, as reported by Martin and Rabineau [246], could be deleterious for the untreated eye. This could be of clinical importance in the management of glaucoma patients, since some authors had recommended a unilateral therapy in glaucoma for some cases [286, 342, 345, 347, 401]. Because part of the local and systemic effects probably result from the vascular β_2 receptor blockage (see below), it should be of interest to repeat this study with a more selective systemic β-blocking agent, such as betaxolol.

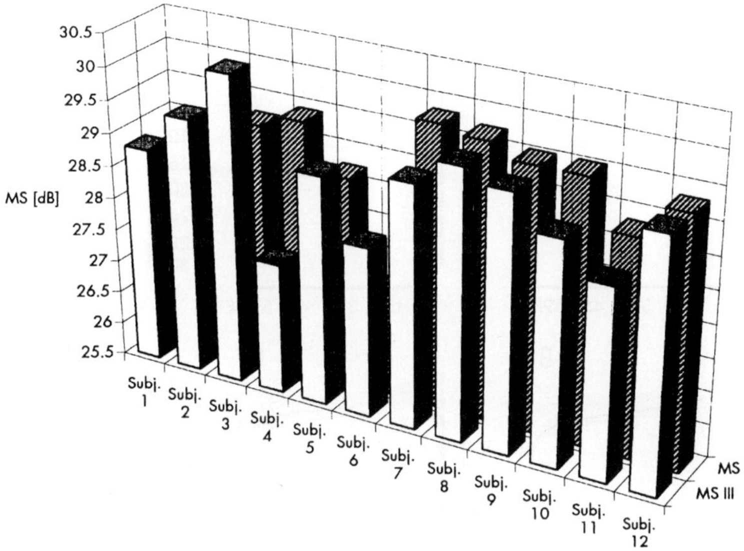

A. Treated Eyes. The mean sensitivity of the first visual fields (MSI), in grey, compared to the third ones (MSIII), in white, shows no significant decrease in 7 normal subjects and no significant increase in 5 others.

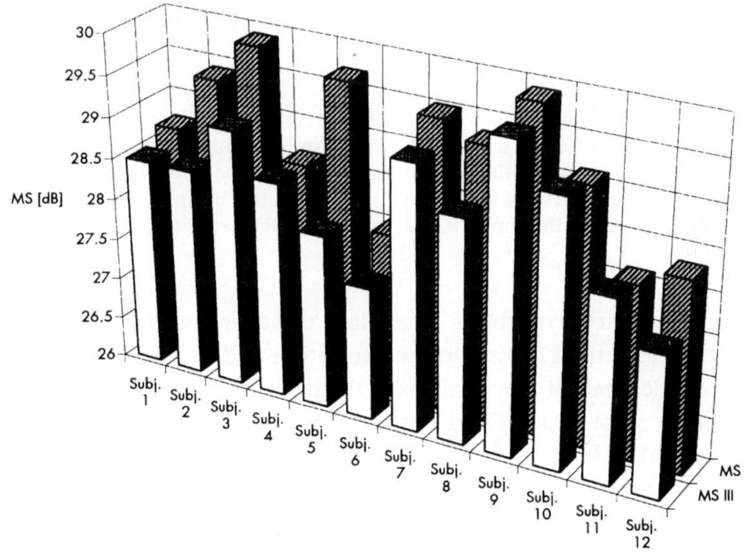

B. Untreated eyes. The mean sensitivity of the third visual fields (MSIII), in white, compared to the first ones (MI), in grey, shows a statistically significant decrease in 10 normal subjects and no changes in 2 others.

Figure 9. Histogram of the mean retinal sensitivity (MS) [dB].

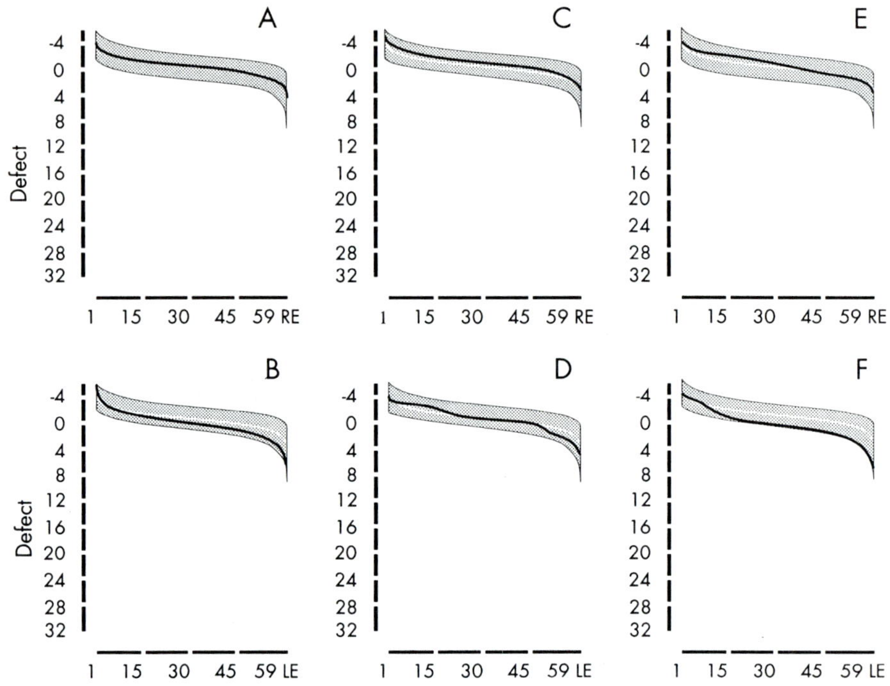

Figure 10. Three cumulative defect curves of subject No 12.
(A) The first cumulative defect curve of the right eye, one week before therapy. (B) The first cumulative defect curve of the left eye, one week before therapy. (C) The second cumulative defect curve of the right eye, one day before therapy. (D) The second cumulative defect curve of the left eye, one day before therapy. (E) The third cumulative defect curve of the right eye, one week after beginning therapy on this eye, with timolol 0.5% twice daily. (F) The third cumulative defect curve of the left eye, one week after beginning therapy on the right eye (contralateral eye), with timolol 0.5% twice daily. (RE = right eye; LE = left eye).

A complementary hypothesis to explain the decrease in retinal sensitivity could be a direct effect of timolol on the retina and more particularly on the serotonergic-dependent mechanisms in the photoreceptor layer, since timolol is known to be a potent antagonist of serotonin [190]. Another mode of action of timolol could be on the NaK-ATPase enzymatic complex in retinal pigment epithelium through serotonin, epinephrin, and norepinephrine antagonism, at the receptor level, for instance, since these biogen amines are known to stimulate NaK-ATPase [397].

Vascular and neural mechanisms could be both involved to explain the decrease of mean retinal sensitivity measured with timolol.

After bilateral instillation of levobunolol 0.5%, Katz et al. [177], using a Humphrey Visual Field Analyzer and program 24–2, found a significant decrease in sensitivity. They suggested that, in normal subjects, generalized, low-level suppression of sensitivity was attained after one drop of levobunolol 0.5%.

(5) Vasoaction of β-Blockers

Only a few studies have been carried out to date on the vasoaction of β-blockers in humans. In one of these, Martin et al. [248, 249, 250] using photographic projection (Fujichrome 100, × 44) measured the retinal vessel diameters before and after instillation of 0.5% timolol twice daily in one eye for 1 week. A total of 12 normal, caucasian subjects aged 25–39 years (average, 30.6 ± 4.2 years) participated in this study. In all, 75% of the subjects had a diminution of retinal arterial size in the treated eye. The mean arterial diametric decrease was 4.1% in treated eyes compared to both untreated eyes and pretreatment values of treated eyes (Fig. 11). These diminutions were statistically significant according to Student's paired t-test ($p < 0.05$). No statistical difference was found among venous diameters (t = 0.065). Results showed that 0.5% timolol may have a vasoconstrictive effect on the retinal arteries of normal human subjects after a week of unilateral instillation twice daily.

Because an optimal method for quantifying vessel diameter changes is presently not available, we tried to use the simplest possible method, viz. the projection of good quality photographs onto a good, fine-grain screen, and made the measurements at least two disc diameters from the optic disc in the same place for every photograph of the same eye. The exact location of the vessel measured was determined by noting its morphology and by measuring the distance to the optic disc. The precision of such measurements was determined by repeatedly (n = 12) measuring vessel diameters as described above from the same site of the same projected image of a normal, healthy human retinal artery at more than 40× magnification. The mean for these measurements was 10.56 ± 0.24 mm. To suppress errors introduced by differences in enlargement between photographs, the measurements were corrected by comparing the distance between the optic disc and foveolar reflex (Fig. 12).

Although Lotmar et al. [50, 219] and Delori et al. [92] developed more sophisticated methods, our method, when correctly used, is certainly no less precise than theirs. Indeed, in the studies of Lotmar and Delori, the vessel diameters were measured in less than 1.5 optic disc diameters – and we know that near the optic disc the retina is 0.56 mm thick compared with only 0.18 mm at its equator [162]. This large thickness of the retina near the optic disc is explained by the nerve fiber layer, since all nerve fibers converge to leave the eye by the optic nerve. Moreover, wall structures and common adventitial sheath-surrounded tissues of arteries and veins [103] are thicker near the optic disc [162], making it difficult to estimate the appearance and the behavior of

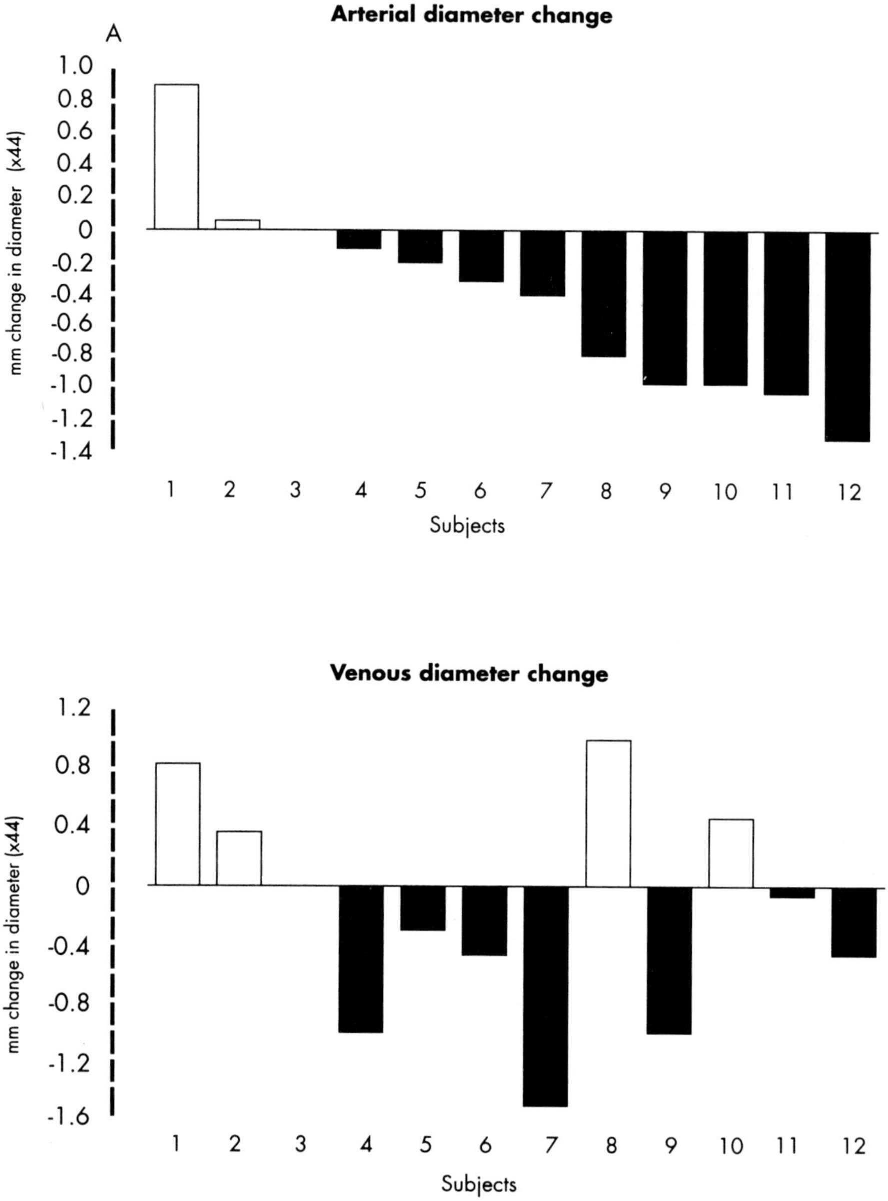

Figure 11. Diameter changes of retinal arteries (A) and veins (B).

Timolol-treated eyes presented a mean decrease in arterial diameter of 0.45 mm (4.1%) that was statistically significant ($p < 0.05$, paired t-test). Diameter changes of veins in timolol-treated eyes were not statistically significant.

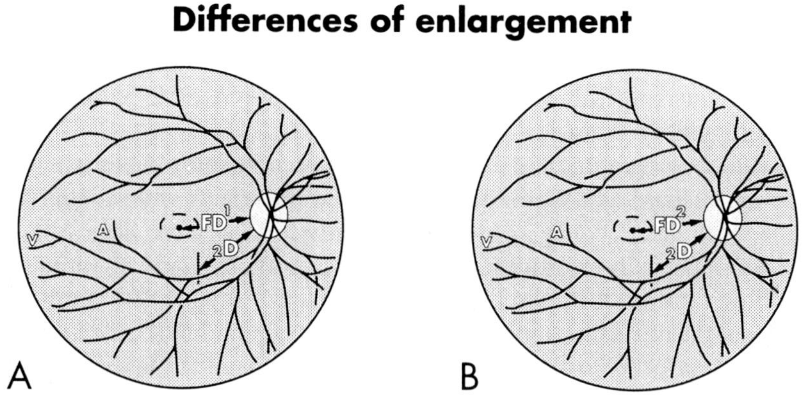

$$\frac{VD\,1 \times FD^2}{FD^1} = \text{corrected VD}$$

Figure 12. Differences of enlargement between photographs were corrected by normalizing the distance between the foveolar reflex and optic disc.
VD, vessel diameter; FD, distance between the foveolar reflex and optic disc; 2D, two diameters of the optic discs; 1, value without timolol; 2 value with timolol; corrected VD, corrected vessel diameter of Photo A with respect to Photo B.

vessels there. We therefore made our measurements at a distance of two optic disc diameters to the disc.

While timolol seems to affect neither blood flow in the anterior eye segment in the rabbit [171] nor dye leakage in fluorescein angiography of the human iris [4], the results of various studies differ as to its effect on blood flow in the posterior eye segment. One hour after administration in the rabbit, L-timolol reduced retinal blood flow by 17% (as measured with laser Doppler velocimetry [394]). However, in the normal human 90 minutes after the instillation of two drops of 0.5% timolol, an average increase in retinal volumetric blood flow of about 13% was measured by the same method [147]. As described by Phillips et al. [306], in the first 1 or 2 hours after the instillation of 0.5% timolol, the drug concentration in aqueous humor was about 150 ng/100 mg, which decreased exponentially. In another study [300], the oxygen tension measured in the cat anterior chamber 90 minutes after 0.5% timolol instillation decreased by 19% (statistically significant). Thus, the relative hypercapnia induced by the hypoxia could perhaps explain the increase of blood flow observed at this time [147].

In an attempt to determine the effect of timolol on optic nerve head autoregulation, visual evoked response/pressure curves were measured in healthy subjects before and after 3 days of 0.5% timolol instilled twice daily in both eyes [307]. Although the ocular perfusion pressures showed a slight though statistically insignificant decrease with timolol, the systemic parameters and the autoregulative behavior did not change [307].

In a videoangiographic and blue-field entoptoscopic study in humans without glaucoma, Richard and Weber [320] compared the effects of 0.5% timolol and 1% pindolol. After being instilled twice daily for 7–9 days, both β-blockers showed a statistically significant negative effect both on nearly all retinal circulation times and on microcirculation in the macular area. These authors concluded that the intrinsic sympathomimetic activity of pindolol could not prevent the negative effect of β-blockers on retinal hemodynamics. On the other hand, Colloton and Perkins [81] reported that timolol dramatically decreased the pulse amplitude in young, healthy volunteers. This decrease in pulse amplitude was so large that it could not be accounted for by the decrease in intraocular pressure, suggesting that timolol decreases intraocular blood flow [81].

Mydriasis is necessary in order to measure retinal blood flow by laser Doppler velocimetry [147] and videoangiography [320]. Tropicamide was used in the first study [230] and cyclopendolate in the second [320]. As used in our study, 5% phenylephrine should not modify the eventual vascular action of timolol. Indeed, although a possible increase in α-adrenoreceptor activity induced by phenylephrine has been reported in essential-hypertension patients who received β-blockers [13, 14], several recent studies [98, 209, 272, 276] have shown that this association did not increase the α-adrenoreceptor activity. Moreover, Mostaghim et al. [272], using ring preparations of rat aortal endothelium, observed a displacement of phenylephrine (an α_1-receptor stimulant with little effect on the β-receptor [385]) with the β-antagonist, timolol. Comparable results were obtained in patients under β-blockers in which the blood pressure did not increase when phenylephrine was infused [98].

Thus, it is possible that timolol acts on both α_1 and β_1-/β_2-receptors. On the other hand, tropicamide and cyclopentolate are anticholinergics that act on α-adrenoreceptors via the muscarinic M_2-receptors [230, 387]. The activation of muscarinic M_2-receptors involves the activation of post-synaptic adrenergic α_2-receptors, which can induce vasoconstriction [387]. The potential vasoactive effects of tropicamide and cyclopentolate in association with β-blockers have yet to be studied. We preferred to use phenylephrine for mydriasis.

Weekers and Collignon-Brach [380] proposed the possibility of a vasoconstrictive action of timolol on retinal vessels, but this has never been observed or measured. The vasoconstriction of retinal arteries that we measured after 7 days of treatment in the treated eyes only is probably the cause of the previously reported decrease in retinal blood flow [81, 320]. Although the opposite might also be true, three explanations for such a decrease can be proposed.

- First, it is well established that the nonselective β-blockers have a direct action on vascular β_2 receptors, causing vasoconstriction [85].
- Second, the blockage of β-receptors in the muscular wall vessel involves a preponderance of α-vasoconstrictive effects [320]. This could explain why the measurements made after acute instillation are different from those made after 1 week of treatment, the time necessary to change the balance in the autonomic nervous system.
- Finally, the decrease in temperature in timolol-treated eyes [389] facilitated the catecholamine vasoconstrictive effect [136].

While the notion of a reduction of intraocular pressure by hypothermia has been variously reported [24, 311, 313], its mechanism of action remains to be elucidated, much as the intimate hypothermic effect of timolol. These three different mechanisms could possibly be implicated in the genesis of the vasoconstrictive effect of timolol.

The fact that retinal vessel changes occurred only in treated eyes suggests that the main ocular effect of timolol is local rather than systemic or central in origin. Moreover, β_1- and β_2-adrenergic receptors were recently found in bovine retinal vessels [121], as were mainly β_2-adrenergic receptors in human retinal vessels [94]. The significant decrease in systemic blood pressure measured by Martin and Rabineau [249] is in agreement with the results of other studies [262, 288]. However, there is probably no relationship between the decrease in systemic blood pressure and retinal arterial vasoconstriction, the latter being evident only in timolol-treated eyes. Therefore, two distinct sites of action for timolol should be involved. According to Neufeld [289, 290], two mechanisms of action for timolol are possible: vasoconstriction, causing a decrease in arterial blood flow; and blockage of ultrafiltrative mechanisms that participate in the formation of aqueous humor. Having shown that the conductivity of the rabbit ciliary epithelium is very low, Brodwall and Fischbarg [54] concluded that the notion of aqueous production by ultrafiltration could not be supported, thus confirming the studies of Bill [35] and Cole [75]. Thus, vasoconstriction seems to be the only valid hypothesis. Since timolol causes vasoconstriction of the retinal arteries as a manifestation of local action, it is conceivable that this effect might cause changes in the ciliary arteries by its action on vascular β_2-receptors [85], resulting in a decrease in arterial blood flow. The measured effect of timolol on retinal vessels suggests that its effect on choroidal circulation and, consequently, on the vasculature of the papilla could be even more marked. This suspected effect of timolol on the ciliary vessels was confirmed by Fahrenbach et al. [117]: Using a microvascular corrosion casting method in rabbits, these authors found that timolol produced a pronounced but localized constriction, whereas betaxolol, a more selective β_1-

blocker, had no significant effect on vascular tone. Several other studies observed similar effects of timolol on the choroidal circulation in experimental animal models [68, 302, 376] and in humans [396].

The role played by the strong vasoconstrictive effect in the lowering of intraocular pressure is discussed below (9, Summary and conclusion on the β-blockers and their possible mechanism of action, p. 66).

(6) β-Blocker Effects on the Cornea Can Help us Understand of the Mechanism of Action of these Drugs

Since some functional similarities exist between corneal epithelium and ciliary epithelium, several mechanisms of action may be very close in both systems.

In a study of 25 patients taking timolol, Van Buskirk [369] found corneal sensitivity was markedly diminished in four elderly patients who had been using the drug for a minimum of three months. In each case, there was restoration of normal corneal sensitivity after discontinuation of timolol. In a comparable study, Spinelli et al. [348] reported remarkably diminished corneal sensitivity in three out of 30 timolol-treated patients. In agreement with Van Buskirk, they reported that timolol maleate appears to have some local anesthetic properties in susceptible individuals and advised monitoring of corneal sensitivity during timolol treatment. Nielsen [293] reported that corneal sensitivity was normal in 65 patients during 9 weeks of timolol treatment. In a study on pigmented rabbits, corneal sensitivity was significantly decreased 10 minutes after a single dose of timolol 0.5% and persisted 1 hour after the last drop of instillation twice daily for 5 days. In other periods, the corneal sensitivity was not significantly increased [264].

The mechanism by which several β-blockers exert a local anesthetic effect remains controversial. The function of corneal epithelium is modulated by the adrenergic system, as indicated in a number of species by the presence of adrenergic corneal nerves [204, 357] and effect of β-adrenergic agonists on both the mitotic rate [131, 265] and the regulation of sodium and chloride transport in corneal epithelium [64, 123]. Moreover, catecholamines [364], particularly dopamine [52] and indoleamines (mainly serotonin [238]), probably play a major role in chloride transport in tears. However, local anesthetic properties of β-blockers are probably nonspecific and independent of β-blockage. One possible mechanism may be the antagonism of timolol against serotonin; indeed, timolol was reported to be a potent antagonist of serotonin stimulation of epithelial chloride transport in the cornea [190]. Moreover, Martin et al. [236] recently measured serotonin, detected in corneal nerves in bovines, in human aqueous humor as well as in tears [238] (see above). If we postulate that corneal serotoninergic nerves or/and the serotonin tear contents are involved in corneal sensitivity, antagonism to β-blockers may play a role in their anesthetic properties. The fact that instillation of serotonin increases the epithelial content of acetylcholine and the corneal sensitivity [373] supports this hypothesis. Furthermore, Nielsen et al. [292] reported that timolol 0.5% increased corneal thickness in both the treated eye and the contralateral control eye. A significantly greater effect was noted in the eye receiving the drug directly. As previously mentioned, Klyce et al. [190] observed that timolol is a potent antagonist to serotonin stimulation of epithelial chloride transport; this mechanism may explain the increase of corneal thickness observed by Nielsen et al. [292] and reciprocally reveal the importance of serotonin in this regulation.

Researchers have identified the local anesthetic or membrane-stabilization effects of β-blockers with their quinidine-like effect [169, 271]. When procaine is administered in combination with propanolol, anesthesia resulting from the former is even antagonized by the latter [1]. On the other hand, lidocaine was reported to have an effect comparable to that of propanolol, both on the intraocular pressure and on corneal anesthesia [275]. However, in contrast to quinidine and propanolol, lidocaine has no significant interaction with the autonomic nervous system [34]. Therefore, although propanolol and lidocaine decrease the intraocular pressure with the same amplitude and both induce a decrease of the sensitivity for 50 minutes, their mechanism of action could be different.

While hypoesthesia following the instillation of β-blocker is usually temporary, seldom lasting more than 10 minutes, there have been some reports of idiosyncratic reactions. Calissendorf [58] reported a case of persistent hypoesthesia during 4 weeks after discontinuation of timolol 0.5%. Other cases of hypoesthesia of unusually long duration have been observed [96]. The relative potency of β-blockers as local anesthetics is variable and has been found to decrease with propanolol, pindolol, and oxyprenolol in decreasing order, respectively, while some have claimed atenolol that shows no anesthetic effect [395]. Variations in physiochemical properties and pharmacokinetic behavior of β-blockers could also be responsible for differences in the topical anesthetic effect [85].

(7) Day/Night Flow of Aqueous Humor and β-Blockers

Following the observation in 1958 by Ericson [114] that the rate of aqueous humor flow follows a circadian cycle, no studies confirmed this until Brubaker's group took on the subject [319]. While Ericson used a suction-cup technique, Reiss et al. [319] and Topper et al. [361] used a fluoro-photometric technique.

The fact that great changes occur naturally (compared to the use of β-blockers or carbonic anhydrase inhibitors) is of considerable interest since up to now the only controllable parameter in glaucoma treatment has been intraocular pressure.

Topper and Brubaker [361] measured the effects of timolol, epinephrine, and acetazolamide on the rate of flow of aqueous humor through the anterior chamber of awake and sleeping human subjects and found that timolol reduced the rate in awake subjects but not in sleeping subjects. These results were confirmed by McCannel et al. [255].

(8) Other Possible Mechanisms of Action of β-Blockers

Colasanti and Trotter [73] observed that timolol has less effect when the eye is pretreated with echothiophate, a relatively irreversible cholinesterase inhibitor. It acts at the ganglionic level, whereas the muscarinic M_2-receptors control the post-synaptic α_2-receptors through the norepinephrine [387]. This suggests that timolol could act partially by activating norepinephrine on the α_2-receptors. That β-blockers may act on another receptor has already been suggested by A. Ungricht and D. Gregory (unpublished data).

(9) Summary and Conclusion on the β-Blockers and their Possible Mechanisms of Action

In an attempt to understand the mechanism of action of β-blockers in decreasing the intraocular pressure in humans, Martin and Rabineau [245, 246, 247, 250] performed several investigations. The effects of timolol were studied on diurnal variations [247], retinal blood vessels [250], systemic blood pressure [250], computerized visual field [245], and serotonin content in aqueous humor [53].

The decrease in amplitude of diurnal variations was 23% in the timolol-treated eyes ($p < 0.01$), with no change found in the contralateral untreated eyes. The diameter of the retinal vessels decreased by 4.1% in the treated eyes ($p < 0.01$; see section 4.2.21 a.5), and no change was measured in the other eyes. The systolic blood pressure decreased by 5.8% ($p < 0.01$). Samples from cataract patients between 8 a.m. and noon showed that the concentration of serotonin decreased by 54% in the aqueous humor of those eyes treated with timolol [53] (Fig. 13).

These results and the fact that

1) timolol has no action on aqueous humor flow during sleep [361],
2) serotonin is an activator of NaK-ATPase [397],
3) indoleamines very probably have a circadian rhythm in human aqueous humor [234, 242],

suggest that the main action of timolol consists of direct or indirect reduction of serotonin stimulation of NaK-ATPase, and that the circadian rhythm of indoleamines drives the circadian rhythm of secretion.

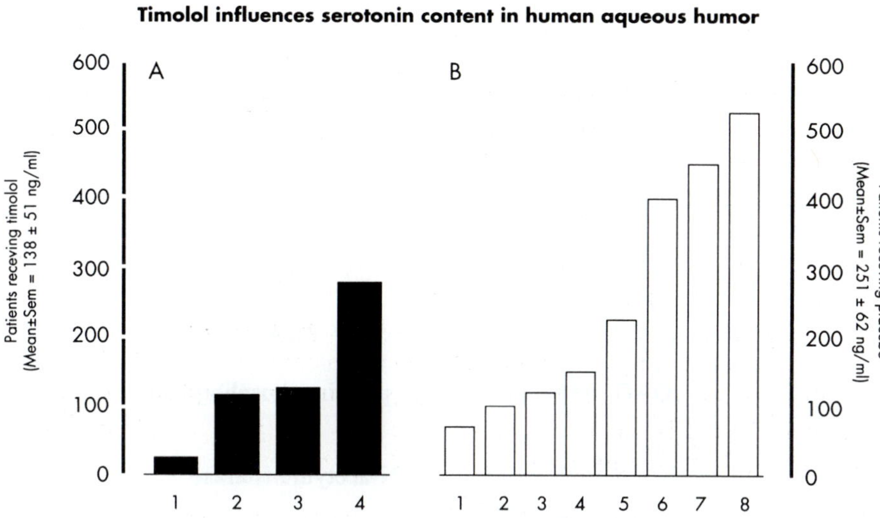

Figure 13. Timolol influences serotonin content in human aqueous humor.
A. Patients receiving timolol. The serotonin concentration was lower in this group (mean ± sem = 138 ± 51 ng/ml).
B. Patients receiving placebo. The serotonin concentration was higher in this group (mean± sem = 251 ± 62 ng/ml).

On the other hand, the local vasoconstrictive effect and the systemic blood pressure decrease produced by β-blockage appear to play complementary roles in the mechanism of action of timolol. What is the importance of this complementary role? As already mentioned, betaxolol, a more selective β_1-blocker, has no effect on the ciliary arteries as opposed to timolol, a non-selective β_1- and β_2-blocker [117, 370]. Therefore, the difference in efficiency between the two drugs could be that part of the action of timolol devoted to vasoconstriction. Since timolol decreases pressure by 33% and betaxolol by 29% [28], the 4% difference could lie in the vasoconstrictive local effect. Expressed in percent of the total effect of timolol, the figure is 12%. Thus, 88% of the timolol effect might result from antagonism with serotonin or serotonin receptors, the remaining 12% being the effect of the vasoconstriction of the ciliary arteries. With regard to the inflow, timolol induces a decrease of 52%, betaxolol of 49.5% [261].

The small difference between hypotensive effects (4%) of timolol and betaxolol, combined with the fact that timolol produces a stenosis of ciliary arteries of 21% whereas betaxolol has no effect, supports the hypothesis that ultrafiltration does not participate in aqueous humor production since vasoconstriction of ciliary arteries has so little effect on the inflow and the intraocular pressure.

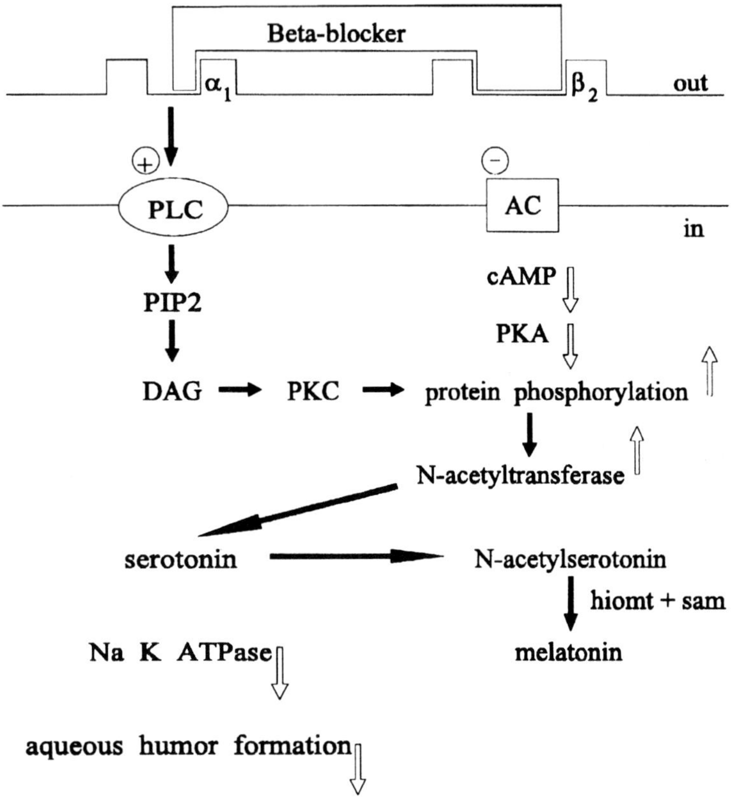

Figure 14. Possible mechanism of action of β-blockers in non-pigmented ciliary epithelium cell.
The β-blocker occupies β_2-receptors giving rise to inhibition of the adenylate cyclase (AC). The β-blocker has also a mild affinity for α_1-receptors. Thus, the activation of phospholipase C (PLC), is produced through α_1-receptor and the inhibition of adenylate cyclase, giving rise to protein phosphorylation increase and N-acetyltransferase formation. Then, serotonin is catabolized by N-acetyltransferase, and the NaK-ATPase no longer stimulated.
α_1 = α_1-receptor; β_2 = β_2-receptor; PIP2 = phosphatidilinositol-4',5'-bisphosphate; DAG = diacylglycerol; PKC = protein kinase C; HIOMT = hydroxyindole-O-methyltransferase; SAM = S-adenosyl-L-methionine; OUT = in posterior chamber; IN = in non-pigmented ciliary epithelium cell; – = inhibition; + = activation.

In conclusion, timolol and probably other β-blockers decrease the intraocular pressure by lowering of the production of aqueous humor through antagonism with serotonin or serotonin receptors. The mechanism could be the following: The β-blocker occupies β_2-receptors and has a mild affinity for α_1-receptors, giving rise to inhibition of adenylate cyclase. Another enzyme, phospholipase C, is activated through the α_1-receptor with help of G proteins, which serve as cellular transducers of the hormone (or drug) signal and give

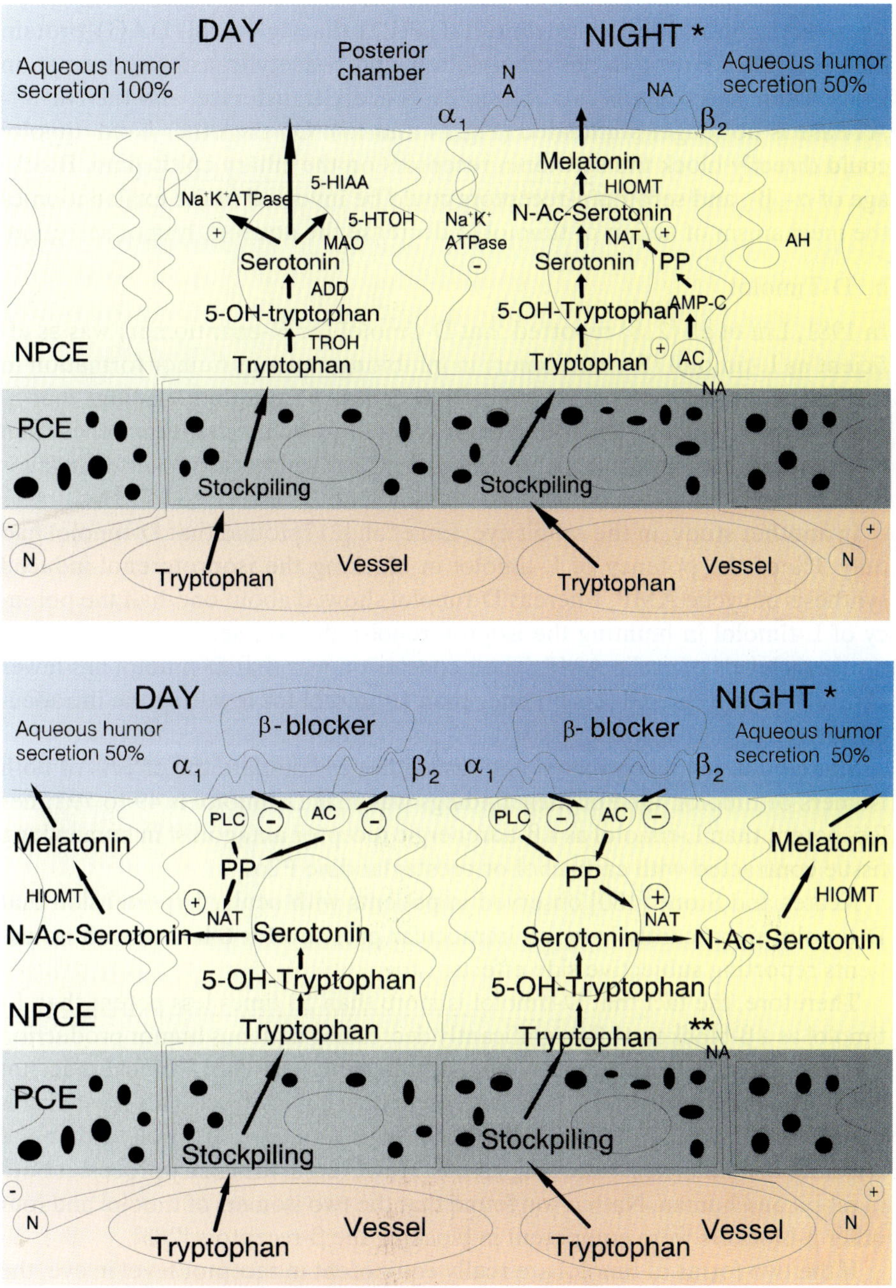

Figure 15. Schematic representation of the possible role of indoleamines in the formation of aqueous humor and the effect of β-blockers on this system. Top, physiological mechanism. Bottom, during β-blocker therapy.

rise to activation of phophatidylinositol (PIP2), diacylglycerol (DAG), protein kinase C (PKC), protein phosphorylation, and N-acetyltransferase formation [244]. Then, serotonin is catabolized by N-acetyltransferase, and the $Na^{+}K^{+}$-ATPase is no longer stimulated (Fig. 14 and 15). On the other hand, timolol could directly block the serotonin receptors on the ciliary epithelium. Blockage of α-, β-, and serotonin-receptors could be involved in the explanation of the mechanism of action of timolol to decrease the aqueous humor secretion.

b. D-Timolol

In 1981, Liu et al. [218] reported that D-timolol (or R-enantiomer) was as efficient as L-timolol (S-enantiomer) in inhibiting aqueous humor formation in the anaesthetized cat eye. Those authors deduced from their findings that timolol might decrease aqueous humor formation by mechanisms other than β-adrenergic blockage, since natural adrenergic receptors are oriented in favor of L-isomers.

In another study, in the rabbit eye, Liu et al. [217] found that D-timolol had only 3% of the potency of L-timolol in blocking the isoproterenol-induced synthesis of cyclic AMP, whereas D-timolol showed about one-half the potency of L-timolol in blunting the isoproterenol-induced rise in iris-ciliary body synthesis levels of cyclic AMP. Their conclusion was that D-timolol has fewer clinical side effects and less potency than L-timolol for lowering the intraocular pressure.

Share et al. [340] conducted various studies to compare the effects of both isomers of timolol. One of their findings was that D-timolol is 49 to 79 times less potent than L-timolol as a β-adrenergic receptor antagonist in human lung tissue contracted with carbachol or prostaglandine F2α.

Keates and Stone [180] observed in patients with ocular hypertension that D-timolol significantly lowered intraocular pressure for 6 hours, with no patients reporting subjective side effects.

Therefore, the fact that D-timolol is more than 50 times less potent than L-timolol as a β-blocker while significantly decreasing aqueous humor production and intraocular pressure seems to support the hypothesis that β-blockers act not only through β-blockage. Yet, the argument may be incorrect: This reasoning is based on the finding that the R-enantiomer of timolol is less potent than the S-isomer in human heart and lung tissues. However, in the ciliary processes both in rabbit and human, Nathanson found that the two isomers of timolol and four other β-blockers were equipotent in blocking the β-receptors [283].

If the two forms of timolol are really equipotent in receptor level in eye, the question is why we continue to use L-timolol, since the D-form seems better tolerated by the patients.

c. Levobunolol

Levobunolol is a β_1- and β_2-blocker without intrinsic sympathomimetic activity like timolol [109].

Several studies on levobunolol 0.5% and 1% compared to timolol 0.5% concluded that the two drugs have the same effects on lowering intraocular pressure, have the same side effects [138, 358, 359], and induce a similar decrease in aqueous humor production [392].

The hypothetical mechanism of action proposed for timolol is likely identical that of levobunolol.

d. Nadolol

In a single-drop application study, Krieglstein [193] found a drop in intraocular pressure between 8 and 11.6 mmHg 3 hours after drug application; the duration of action was between 6 hours and 9 hours with concentrations of 0.3% to 2%. Compared to timolol, nadolol and diacetyl nadolol are less efficient if the intraocular pressure-lowering and duration properties are taken into account, both in normal subjects and in patients with ocular hypertension or glaucoma [108, 110, 194].

e. Metipranolol

Metipranolol is a non-selective β_1 and β_2-blocker without intrinsic sympathomimetic activity and with little membrane-stabilizing effect. Metipranolol is metabolized in the eye by nonspecific esterase in desacetyl-metipranolol (DMP). This metabolite has about the same effect as the mother-substance.

Like the other β-blockers, metipranolol can cause corneal anaesthesia [95].

B. β-Blockers with Intrinsic Sympathomimetic Activity (with ISA)

a. Pindolol

Pindolol is linked to the names of Bonomi and Steindler, who published the first study on this nonselective β-blocker in 1975 [49]. Moreover, these authors suggested that pindolol acts by inhibiting aqueous humor production, because no significant variation in the outflow facility was observed. Endowed with intrinsic sympathomimetic activity, pindolol is slightly less potent than timolol in decreasing intraocular pressure in the rabbit [47] and probably equipotent with timolol in humans [11, 87].

In an interesting study, Flammer and coworkers [126] investigated the influence of pindolol and timolol treatment on the visual fields of glaucoma patients. After 6 months of treatment, the pindolol-treated group showed a slight tendency towards improvement in their visual fields, the timolol-treated group revealing a very slight tendency towards deterioration. The authors concluded that the two drugs, which both reduced intraocular pressure, did not necessarily have the same effect on visual function. We can add that the pressure-lowering mechanism could not be exactly the same for the two drugs.

b. Carteolol and Befunolol

Since both drugs have intrinsic sympathomimetic activity, they are also discretely less potent than timolol. Carteolol was first synthesized and investigated in Japan [287]. The controversy concerning the systemic effects began with the first publications: Kitazawa et al. [189] found a decrease in pulse rate and systemic blood pressure, whereas Horie et al. [164] found no changes in systemic blood pressure and resting pulse rate.

In a comparison of ocular and cardiovascular effects of carteolol 2% and timolol 0.5%, Brazier et al. [51] found that the two agents appeared comparable with regard to ocular hypotensive and cardiovascular effects, whereas Scoville et al. [334] observed that significantly fewer patients in the group treated with carteolol reported adverse systemic events (specifically: eye irritation). Thus, some question persists about the intrinsic sympathomimetic activity of this agent.

Like carteolol, befunolol was developed in Japan [356]. Similar to carteolol, befunolol seems able to produce blepharitis in some patients [280, 335]. In morphological studies of the effect of subconjunctival administration and instillation of befunolol as well as instillation of timolol on the ciliary epithelium in rabbit, Nishimura et al. [297] and Hiramatsu et al. [155, 156, 157] observed a swelling of mitochondria and suggested a relationship between these morphological changes and a pharmacological mechanism for lowering intraocular pressure.

Befunolol and timolol (but not pilocarpine) have been shown to inhibit the phagocytosis of cultured retinal pigment epithelium from the chick embryo at the level used in clinical practice [252]. The clinical relevance of these interesting findings warrants further investigation.

4.2.2.2 β_1-Blockers

a. Betaxolol

Ever since the kinetic studies of Nathanson [283] it is known that betaxolol, usually considered a β_1-adrenergic-selective antagonist, is relatively nonselective in the ciliary processes. Indeed, the heart/ciliary processes potency ratio was 1.1 for betaxolol and 1.2 for timolol.

On the other hand, according to Nathanson [284], betaxolol is useful in patients because it is considerably less potent than timolol (Ka = 150 nM versus 5 nM for timolol). As such, enough gets into the eye to block ocular β-receptors, but the amount absorbed systemically is less able to block systemic β-receptors.

According to the fluorophotometric and tonographic study of Reiss and Brubaker [318], betaxolol suppressed aqueous humor flow without the consistent effect on outflow resistance found with timolol.

Clinically important are the findings of Collignon-Brach [77, 78] that compared to timolol betaxolol produces long-term improvement of the visual field, confirming the findings of Demailly [93]. Martin and Rabineau, on the other hand, revealed vasoconstriction of human retinal arteries under timolol treatment, results confirmed by Yoshida and coworkers [396]; Collignon and coworkers [76] found a relaxation under betaxolol in human retinal arteries.

b. Atenolol

Atenolol is considered a selective β_1 adrenergic antagonist without intrinsic sympathomimetic activity [111] and without membrane-stabilizing properties [386]. Collignon-Brach [79] and Sterk [351] observed tachyphylaxis with atenolol 4%. Ros et al. [326] compared the ocular penetration of atenolol, timolol, propanolol, and metoprolol. These authors discovered poor ocular penetration for atenolol, something they attributed to the low lipophilicity of this agent. Finally, a duration of action of 6 hours [386], a pulse-rate reduction [350], and a slight depressive effect on blood pressure [299] prevented atenolol from being used clinically.

c. Metoprolol

Also considered a selective β_1 adrenergic antagonist without intrinsic sympathomimetic activity, metoprolol (both isomers L and D) seems more selective than betaxolol. Indeed, whereas most β-blockers have a higher absolute affinity for ciliary process receptors than for cardiac receptors, metoprolol is the exception and seems to have a *lower affinity* for the β_2-receptors than for the β_1-receptors [283].

If this is the case, the mechanism of decrease of aqueous humor formation could be different from that of timolol or betaxolol, or as already mentioned the blockage of β_2-receptors could not be the main action of β-blockers.

Collignon-Brach and Weekers [80], in a comparative study between metoprolol 3% and timolol 0.5%, concluded that both timolol and metoprolol decreased intraocular pressure by reducing aqueous humor secretion without increasing facility of outflow. The two agents had similar short- and long-term efficacy, which did not diminish even after several months of use. When blocking β_2-receptors, timolol causes marked constriction of bronchi and of peripheral vessels. Hence, it is contraindicated in bronchial asthma and ischemic optic neuropathy. This is not the case with metoprolol, which does not block β_2-receptors.

Metoprolol 1% was found to reduce the intraocular pressure by 23%, and concentrations of 2%, 4%, and 8% were no more efficient than that of 1% [57]. In an interesting study, Palkama and coworkers [301] compared the effects of adrenergic agonists and α- and β-antagonists on intraocular pressure and adenylate cyclase activity in the ciliary processes of the rabbit. In normotensive eyes, agonist isoproterenol (β) and antagonists labetolol (α and β), metoprolol (β_1), and acebutolol (β_1) decreased intraocular pressure significantly. In hypertensive eyes, only isoproterenol and labetolol decreased intraocular pressure markedly. Timolol (β_1 and β_2) did not decrease intraocular pressure, although it did inhibit adenylate cyclase activity as actively as labetalol. The other antagonists showed no inhibitory effect in this respect. For these authors, the results indicated that α-activity (labetalol, α and β) seems to potentiate the β-activity (timolol, β_1 and β_2) in decreasing intraocular pressure. Similarly, metoprolol (β_1), without affecting adenylate cyclase activity, decreased intraocular pressure as well. Though the notion of receptor duplicity already described above (Point 8: Other Possible Mechanisms of Action of β-Blockers) seems obvious here, the role of adenylate cyclase in the mechanism of action of β-blockers remains unclear.

4.2.2.3 β_2-Blockers

a. Butoxamine

Butoxamine is a relatively selective β_2-antagonist. It blocks β_2 vasodilator and other smooth muscle inhibitory effects of isoproterenol [384]. In a study on the suppression of ocular hypertension induced by water loading in the rabbit, Rowland and Potter [328] found that the β_2-antagonist, butoxamine, and the β_1-antagonist, metoprolol, were ineffective in lowering the artificially elevated intraocular pressure, in contrast to β_2-agonists, which were very effective.

4.2.3 Second Messenger Activators

4.2.3.1 Adenylate Cyclase Activators

a. Forskolin

Forskolin is a labdane diterpenoid that was extracted from the root of the plant *Coleus forskohlii Briq* in 1977 by Baht et al. [30]. Forskolin stimulates adenylate cyclase activity without interaction with cell-surface receptors, increasing intracellular c-AMP levels and decreasing aqueous humor production [63]. The hypotensive effect of forskolin was lower in pigmented than in albino rabbits, although duration was longer, perhaps because forskolin has specific affinity towards melanin granules [341]. Bartels et al. [20] investigated the effect of topical forskolin in rabbits on intraocular pressure and aqueous humor formation using pneumatonometry and fluorophotometry. Forskolin produced a prolonged 10-fold reduction of intraocular pressure and decreased humor formation with increased cyclic AMP concentration in aqueous humor. Moreover, the same authors, using forskolin in combination with epinephrine, recorded a decrease in intraocular pressure of longer duration than under separate administration of either 0.1% epinephrine or 1% forskolin. The latter findings support the preceding data of Jumblatt and North [173], that forskolin and cyclic AMP potentiate the sympathetic neurosecretion in the rabbit iris/ciliary body.

Forskolin did not significantly decrease intraocular pressure in the monkey after the second day of treatment [205, 207].

In humans, although acute forskolin instillation induces a decrease of the aqueous humor formation and intraocular pressure [208, 374], it seems [309] that forskolin is not a promising agent for glaucoma therapy because of rapid development of tachyphylaxis.

b. Calcium-Channel Blockers

Instillation of verapamil elevates aqueous-humor c-AMP levels in rabbits [22, 336], as do β-blockers. Moreover, verapamil blocks the slow channel, thereby preventing the entrance of calcium into the cell [285], whereas c-AMP increases the slow channel current [257]. These contradictory effects of verapamil could explain the elevation of intraocular pressure some authors observed in rabbits and humans [22]. However, a decrease of intraocular pressure has also been reported in humans following administration of calcium channel blockers [146, 270]. This inconsistency is perplexing and remains unexplained.

4.2.3.2 Calcium Ion (Ca^{2+})

The calcium ion (Ca^{2+}) is able to activate adenylate cyclase in rabbit ciliary process membranes by taking action on another enzyme used by forskolin [363]. Since calcium ion or calmodulin-binding calcium activates the adenylate cyclase, producing an increase in c-AMP which in turn activates the slow channel (that is, the entrance of calcium into the cell), another mechanism must exist that regulates the entrance of Ca^{2+} into the cell. As far as we know, no study has concerned the effects of Ca^{2+} on intraocular pressure.

4.2.4 Serotonin Inhibitor

a. Ketanserine

Ketanserine was first synthesized in 1977, and it is the prototype of a new series of serotoninergic antagonists. This substance blocks the 5-HT_2-receptors competitively and selectively without significant effect on the 5-HT_1-receptors [371]. Moreover, ketanserine is able to block some α_1-receptors and has some affinity for histamine H1 receptors as well [170].

Chang et al. [65] observed that the ocular hypotensive effect of ketanserine was markedly attenuated in sympathectomized rabbits and concluded that this agent acted primarily by antagonizing the action of norepinephrine on α_1 adrenoreceptors. These results can be compared with those of Cohen et al. [71], who found that, although ketanserin decreased blood pressure in hypertensive rats, a more selective 5-HT_2 antagonist (LY538657), which showed minimal affinity for vascular α adrenergic receptors, did not lower blood pressure in these animals. This indicates that blockage of both central and vascular serotonin receptors is not a sufficient mechanism to lower blood pressure in this model of hypertension. Moreover, LY53857 at doses sufficient to eliminate 5-HT_2-receptor activation did not enhance blood-pressure reduction produced by the α-adrenergic receptor antagonist, phentolamine, in normotensive or spontaneously hypertensive rats [72]. Thus, although it is not known whether or not LY53857 has an effect on the intraocular pressure, it is interesting to establish a correspondence between the findings of Chang et al. and Cohen et al., and to hypothesize than serotonin, which probably plays a role in aqueous humor dynamics, does not act through 5-HT_2-receptors but perhaps through 5-HT_1, since methysergide, a 5-HT_1-receptor antagonist, inhibits the peak rise of intraocular pressure in acute irritative response to topical neutral formaldehyde 1% in the rabbit eye [197].

In a study of the effects of serotonin and ketanserin on intraocular pressure in the rabbit, Krootila et al. [196] found that topical 2% serotonin decreased the intraocular pressure by 4 mmHg in normal eyes, whereas intracameral injection of serotonin caused a rise in the intraocular pressure and a breakdown of the blood-aqueous barrier, both effects of which were not inhibited by sympathectomy. On the other hand, topical 2% ketanserine lowered the intraocular pressure by 4 mmHg. This hypotensive action was inhibited after sympathectomy. Therefore, the hypotensive actions of topical serotonin and ketanserin on intraocular pressure seem dependent on the intact sympathetic innervation of the eye for ketanserin, but not for serotonin. The blockage of α_1 receptor therefore seems to be the mechanism through which ketanserin lowers intraocular pressure.

The ocular hypotensive action of ketanserin in rabbit was confirmed by Conway et al. [82].

Finally, it is interesting to notice that clomipramine, a potent and rather selective blocker of serotonin transport [16], when used in a daily dose of 50 mg per os, decreased intraocular pressure and its diurnal variations significantly in humans (Martin XD, 1983, unpublished data).

4.2.5 Na^+K^+-ATPase Inhibitors

a. Ouabaine

Ouabain or strophantin-G is a cardiac glycoside derived from *Strophanthus gratus Squill* [160]. First investigated by Cole [74] in the rabbit and Simon et al. [344] in the cat, the Na^+K^+-ATPase mechanism was observed by Riley [321] to be linked with glycolysis in the ciliary epithelium and inhibited by ouabaine. Since these original studies on ouabain, the interest in this substance has waned.

b. Vanadate

Becker [25], in his Proctor Lecture entitled "Vanadate and Aqueous Humor Dynamics," summarized the contemporary knowledge of 1980 as follows:

> "Topical administration of 0.5% vanadate lowers intraocular pressure in monkey and rabbit. This appears to be a result of a reduction in the rate of aqueous humor secretion, probably resulting from the inhibition of ciliary epithelium membrane Na^+K^+-ATPase. The ubiquitous vanadate and its interactions with catecholamines and ascorbate may play a role in regulating the sodium pump of the ciliary epithelium. Adrenergic blocking agents may also lower intraocular pressure by inhibiting the Na^+K^+-ATPase of the ciliary epithelium."

Ten years later, while the adrenergic blocking agents do appear to act indirectly on Na^+K^+-ATPase [231, 237], the ocular hypotensive effect of vanadate would appear to more likely act on other cellular mechanisms. Indeed, Mittag et al. [268] found that at the time of lowered intraocular pressure the vanadate content in iris and ciliary body in the rabbit was too short to inhibit a significant fraction of Na^+K^+-ATPase or to cause a significant stimulation of adenylate cyclase. Other studies confirmed the decrease in aqueous humor flow without significant effect on outflow facility [310]. Moreover, topical vanadate did not alter anterior chamber aqueous humor protein or cyclic AMP [198]. In a study on the mechanism of action of vanadate in the rabbit, Delamere and Williams [91] found that vanadate could act through adrenergic mechanisms to lower intraocular pressure.

c. 12-R-HETE

See Section 4.4.3.3 Cytochrome P450-Dependent Pathway (p. 89).

4.3 Drugs Acting on the Outflow System

4.3.1 Cholinergics

a. Pilocarpine

Since Hardy's discovery of this alkaloid present in *Pilocarpus pennatifolius* [150] in 1875, and since its first use in glaucoma treatment by Weber [378] one year thereafter, pilocarpine has become the most-used and studied miotic.

Pilocarpine has three different main actions:

1) It produces a miosis and stimulates accommodation.
2) It increases the facility of outflow of the aqueous humor. This effect seems secondary to the displacement of the scleral spur and, consequently, to the change of the trabecular meshwork configuration, according to Kaufman and Bárány [178, 179], who found a loss of acute pilocarpine effect on outflow facility following surgical disinsertion and retro-displacement of the ciliary muscle from the scleral spur in the cynomolgus monkey.
3) It reduces the uveoscleral flow of aqueous humor [39].

Pilocarpine acts both on muscarinic M_1- and M_2-receptors [40, 144, 149, 224, 387]. Moreover, the neuronal control of α_2-adrenoreceptors is mediated by ganglionic M_2-receptors (Fig. 16) [387]. Therefore, pilocarpine acts upon the M_2-receptors in the iris sphincter and ciliary muscle, and on M_1-receptors at the ganglionic level. This probably explains systemic side effects such as arterial hypotension, bradycardia, and nausea [152, 230, 387]. Pilocarpine has also been shown indirectly to produce arterial vasoconstriction by means of neuronal control of α_2-adrenergic receptors mediated by ganglionic M_2-receptors [387]. This may explain the reduction of aqueous humor formation sometimes reported in studies on pilocarpine [18, 263].

b. Aceclidine

Étienne [115] reported that aceclidine (3-acetoxyquinuclidine) was synthesized in the USSR in 1960 by Rubtizov and Michlina and used for the first time as a miotic by Mashkovski and Zaitzeva.

Aceclidine activates muscarinic receptor and shows weak anticholinesterase activity [97, 116, 213, 324]. Therefore, aceclidine is both a direct and an indirect parasympathomimetic agent. While the miotic effect is slightly less marked

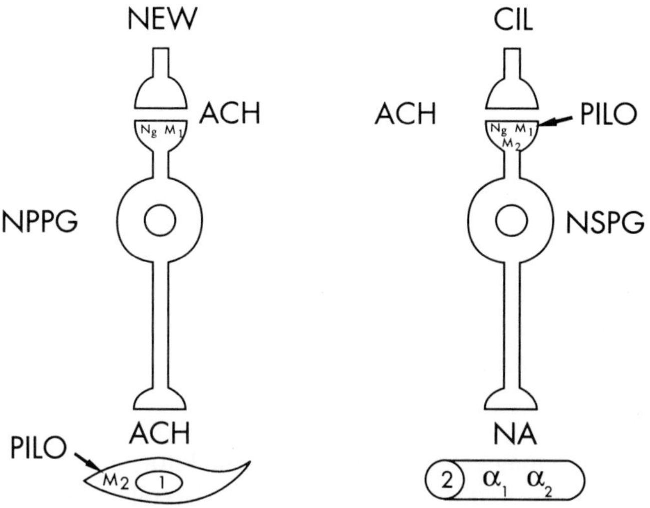

Figure 16. Action sites of pilocarpine. After instillation, pilocarpine acts mainly on M_2-muscarinic receptors of the iris sphincter and can have systemic effects through its action on the M_1-ganglionic muscarinic receptors.
NEW = Edinger-Westphal nucleus; CIL = sympathetic intermediolateral group of the spinal cord; ACH = acetylcholine; PILO = pilocarpine; NPPG = postganglionic parasympathetic neuron; NSPG = postganglionic sympathetic neuron; NA = norepinephrine; NG = ganglionic nicotinic receptor; M_1 = type-1 muscarinic receptor; M_2 = type-2 muscarinic receptor; α_1 = α_1 postsynaptic adrenergic receptor; α_2 = α_2 postganglionic adrenergic receptor; 1 = smooth muscle cell of the iris sphincter; 2 = vascular wall.

than that of pilocarpine and intraocular pressure-lowering is comparable, the amount of accommodation effected is much less with aceclidine (0.3–0.7 diopters after aceclidine 2% versus 2.3–6 diopters after pilocarpine 2% in emmetropic subjects) [118, 308], and the reduction of the anterior chamber depth is less than that with pilocarpine [122, 128, 129]. However, idiosyncratic reaction can occurs with aceclidine, as observed in a glaucoma patient who presented 8 diopters accommodation after one drop aceclidine 2% as well as when exposed in strong light (Martin, unpublished observation).

This dissociation between accommodative and outflow facility functions, usually observed with aceclidine, led Erickson-Lamy and Schroeder [113] to investigate these in vivo in the cynomolgus monkey eye. While the accommodation was limited to an average of 5 diopters with aceclidine, the accommodative ability was 19 diopters with pilocarpine. These authors concluded that the accommodative and outflow facility functions of ciliary muscle were dissociated, suggesting several subpopulations of muscarinic receptors in the ciliary muscle. Finally, since the blockage of uveo-scleral outflow by pilocarpine appears to be secondary to the contraction of ciliary muscle, which obliterates the spaces between the muscle bundles, it is of interest to consider that this might not be the case with aceclidine [38, 241].

c. Carbachol

Like aceclidine, carbachol is also both a direct and an indirect parasympathomimetic agent. More potent than pilocarpine, carbachol has the same side effects and, as does pilocarpine, may cause an important forward displacement of lens with the risk of an angle-closure glaucoma in eyes with shallow anterior chamber [129].

Presently, carbachol is used topically or intracamerally to control intraocular pressure after cataract extraction [163, 214, 317].

d. Echothiophate

Echothiophate is a long-acting cholinesterase inhibitor, still used today in certain glaucomas associated with aphakia. Lütjen-Drecoll and Kaufman investigated its mode of action from a morphological point of view [221] in cynomolgus monkey eyes after long-term topical treatment. The echothiophate-treated eyes exhibited increased intraocular pressure, collapse, and densification of the trabecular meshwork with accumulation of extracellular material in the cribriform region, alterations in the shape and orientation of Schlemm's canal and the ciliary muscle, and discontinuities between ciliary muscle bundles and trabecular beams. Those authors concluded that the structural alterations observed were mediated in part by anterior segment muscarinic receptors, that mechanical factors and underperfusion of the meshwork were involved, and that the echiothiophate had no direct toxic effect. These observations might explain the disappearance of effect sometimes met by patients chronically treated with echiothiophate [191]. On the other hand, clinical practice teaches us that after discontinued therapy, the responsiveness to echothiophate can be restored, perhaps because these alterations are not totally irreversible.

4.4 Drugs Acting on Outflow and/or Inflow Systems

4.4.1 α-Adrenergic Stimulators

a. Epinephrine or Adrenaline

Epinephrine stimulates both α- and β-adrenergic receptors. In 1966, Sears proposed that topical epinephrine exerts three previously suggested effects upon the maintenance level of intraocular pressure in glaucoma patients [335]. First, as Goldmann's study showed [143], there is a decrease of aqueous humor production. Second, according to studies by Becker and Weekers, there is an immediate increase in outflow facility [26, 382]. Third, as Ballintine showed, there may be an increase in outflow facility lasting several weeks or months [17]. Whereas the first two mechanisms seem well established, the third remains hypothetical. Its mechanism has been related to the metabolism of glycosaminoglycans in the trabecular meshwork [337]. However, it could be due simply to the removal of the blockage of uveoscleral flow, since it is seen in groups of patients previously under cholinergic therapy.

Since the studies of Bhattacherjee et al. in rabbits [31] and Camras et al. [60] in humans on the inhibitory effect of indomethacin – one of the most potent inhibitors of the prostaglandin-forming cyclooxygenase [127] – on the hypotensive action of epinephrine, it seems that the main action of epinephrine, namely, reducing intraocular pressure, is achieved by stimulating endogenous prostaglandin synthesis [61]. Another cyclo-oxygenase inhibitor, piroxicam, which, unlike indomethacin, does not block Ca^{2+} movements, also blocks the epinephrine-induced rise in outflow facility [10].

Recently, Camras and Podos [62], in a review of the relevant literature, concluded that several medical and laser treatment methods presently used in glaucoma therapy reduced intraocular pressure, at least in part by stimulating endogenous prostaglandin synthesis. Their conclusion was based on four lines of evidence:

1) Certain prostaglandins are potent ocular hypotensive agents;
2) adrenergic and cholinergic agonists stimulate prostaglandin synthesis by ocular tissues in vitro;
3) epinephrine and argon-laser trabeculoplasty (ALT) cause elevation of prostaglandin levels in the aqueous humor in vivo;
4) prostaglandin-synthesis inhibitors, such as indomethacin or flurbiprofen, block or partially inhibit the reduction of intraocular pressure produced by epinephrine, para-aminoclonidine, forskolin, vanadate, verapamil, arachidonic acid, and argon laser trabeculoplasty in rabbits, cats, monkeys, and humans.

Finally, those authors emphasized that, because several drugs as well as aspirin and indomethacin are very frequently used for many different purposes, it was of clinical importance to be assured that patients with glaucoma therapy had not taken prostaglandin inhibitors that might interfere with the efficacy of their primary treatment.

b. Dipivefrin

In 1975, McClure [256] introduced a new substance, dipivalyl epinephrine (DPE) or dipivefrin. This agent is an analog of epinephrine in which two pivalic acid groups are added to epinephrine. This chemical change confers upon dipivefrin more lipophilicity and, consequently, improved penetration through the cornea. The bioavailability of the drug is thus higher and the necessary amount of substance lower in comparison to epinephrine.

The first studies with dipivefrin showed that its ability to decrease intraocular pressure and its side effects were comparable to those of epinephrine [41, 174]. However, in studies performed more recently, dipivefrin was found to have less marked cardiovascular side effects than epinephrine [184].

Dipivefrin is a prodrug of epinephrine which is hydrolyzed to epinephrine and pivalic acid, mainly in the cornea [9]. Pivalic acid, which enhances the ocular penetration of dipivefrin, is more rapidly eliminated from the eye than the pharmacologically active portion of the molecule, and studies of corneal tissues have shown that pivalic acid has no toxic effects in vivo and is mildly toxic to endothelial cells in culture only at high concentrations [349], while raising the corneal penetration by 17-fold [2, 226].

c. Guanethidine

Guanethidine is an adrenergic neuron-blocking agent that acts at postganglionic adrenergic nerve endings principally by depletion of norepinephrine from the nerve fiber [384], which blocks the neural release of the transmitter and prevents its re-uptake into neuronal stores [253, 254]. Its chronic administration gives rise to a greater supersensitivity of effector cells for norepinephrine than for epinephrine; this occurs after 2 weeks [384].

Used in glaucoma patients since the beginning of the 1960s [200], guanethidine lowers intraocular pressure probably by reducing aqueous humor production and perhaps by eliciting a transient increase of outflow facility [46, 48]. The supersensitivity induced by guanethidine enhances the hypotensive effect on intraocular pressure of epinephrine. Thus, the combination of the two drugs is more potent than either guanethidine or epinephrine alone [158, 274, 366]. This association was also reported to be equipotent with pilocarpine 1% [325] and timolol 0.5% [154]. In glaucomatous eyes, however, Hoyng and Dake [165] measured a biphasic response of intraocular pressure with a 36% increase in aqueous humor production during the hypertensive phase occurring between 1 and 3 hours after instillation of a mixture of guanethidine 3% and adrenaline 0.5%. These authors attributed this event to a transient disruption of the blood-aqueous barrier induced by the release of prostaglandins.

d. Norepinephrine or Noradrenaline

First used in 1954 by Hofmann [161] as a topical solution on glaucomatous eyes, it was noticed that norepinephrine penetration through the cornea was limited by its high polarity and low liposolubility. For this reason, norepinephrine dipivalylate, a prodrug analog of norepinephrine, was developed and administered to ocular hypertensive patients, a significant lowering effect occurring with a 0.5% concentration. Of interest was the slow onset of hypotensive effect 4 hours after instillation and the prolonged effect during the 8 ensuing hours [352].

According to Pollack [312, 314], the mechanisms of action of epinephrine and norepinephrine are similar, both of which produce an increase in outflow facility.

While the main action of norepinephrine seems to be the same as that of epinephrine, no study is available about the possible stimulation of prostaglandin synthesis by norepinephrine. Interactions between norepinephrine and prostaglandins, however, have been known since Duffin et al. [99] found that flubiprofen, a potent cyclooxygenase inhibitor, suppressed the development of subsensitivity with norepinephrine or adrenergic adaptation in rabbit eyes.

The role and the mechanism of action of norepinephrine in aqueous humor dynamics is probably major, though still not well understood. The difficulty could lie in the fact that the β-adrenergic mechanism predominates in humans, whereas the α-adrenergic mechanism predominates in some other species [137]. The difference in the effects of β-blockers on the intraocular pressure in the rabbit and humans probably stems from the different adrenergic balance between α- and β-receptors in these two species.

Finally, the possible activating effect of norepinephrine on the N-acetyltransferase recently found in the human iris/ciliary body [244] warrants further investigation.

e. Clonidine and Apraclonidine

Clonidine and apraclonidine are both α-adrenergic agonists capable of reducing intraocular pressure. The use of clonidine, on the other hand, is limited by these adverse systemic effects, particularly that of blood-pressure reduction [159]. Although several articles have attempted to demonstrate a central mechanism of action of clonidine in lowering intraocular pressure through the stimulation of central α-adrenoceptors [166, 167, 168], the mechanism remains uncertain until now.

According to Wang et al. [375], apraclonidine seems to effect less systemic blood pressure reduction than does clonidine. The intraocular pressure-lowering effect of apraclonidine could be mediated through the activation of the α_2-adrenergic receptors, which occur predominantly in the ciliary processes [269]; these, in turn, give rise to an increase in endogenous prostaglandin synthesis [375]. This hypothesis is based on the observations that the levels of prostaglandins F2α and E2 were increased in both eyes after unilateral apraclonidine instillation in rabbit, and that flurbiprofen completely blocked the hypotensive effect of apraclonidine in the monkey. In glaucoma patients, however, the same authors found no inhibition of the reduction of intraocular pressure using flurbiprofen [375]. If the stimulation of endogenous synthesis of prostaglandins, particularly that of prostaglandin F2α, known to increase the uveoscleral outflow, can explain a part of the action of this drug, another parameter, such as the vasoconstrictive effect, must be taken into consideration. Indeed, Fahrenbach et al. [117] measured an intense vasoconstriction of 37% on the ciliary arteries in the rabbit eye after unilateral instillation of apraclonidine. This effect was stronger than that of phenylephrine (28%) or of timolol (21%).

Recently, Lish and co-workers [215] reported an additive effect of 1% apraclonidine for intraocular pressure in patients already receiving combined therapy with timolol and acetazolamide. This observation is interesting and suggests that timolol does not act on the α_2 receptors. Moreover, apraclonidine reduces the intraocular pressure during sleep, contrary to timolol [277]. Therefore, the α_2-receptors probably do not play a role in the circadian variations of intraocular pressure, whereas β_2 receptors and serotonin receptors do.

In humans, apraclonidine induces a follicular conjunctivitis in 26% to 36% of the cases, which constitutes a serious limitation for its chronic use [227, 277].

f. Pargyline

Pargyline is a selective monoamine-oxidase-inhibitor-B (MAO-B) [32] found to lower intraocular pressure in the rabbit probably by means of a reduction of the rate of aqueous humor formation without a change in the outflow facility [398]. The hypotensive effect was also observed with pargyline 0.5% in glaucoma patients [258].

Of interest are the observations of Zeller et al. [399], who noticed that reserpine, a drug that depletes stores of catecholamines and serotonin, decreased intraocular pressure by reducing aqueous humor production, and that this action was slightly counteracted by a small drop in the facility of outflow in the rabbit eye. Moreover, when reserpine was instilled together with pargyline, aqueous humor formation was extremely low. From these data, the authors suggested that, although the action of reserpine or pargyline on aqueous humor dynamics was quite similar, their mechanisms of action must be different.

Therefore, both reserpine and pargyline interfere with indoleamines: reserpine with the storage of serotonin, and pargyline by blockage of the degradation of 5-methoxytryptamine to 5-methoxyindolacetaldehyde [135].

Although in rat primary astrocyte cultures serotonin oxidation to 5-hydroxyindoleacetic acid seems to be carried out principally by MAO-A [124] and in mice brain [133] by pargyline, a MAO-B inhibitor causes some inhibition of MAO-A as well in these two conditions.

In summary, pargyline acts on two different levels in the metabolism of indoleamines. First, it partially inhibits the oxydation of serotonin to 5-hydroxyindoleacetic acid, and second it blocks the degradation of 5-methoxytryptamine to 5-methoxyindolacetaldehyde. Therefore, it favors the melatonin pathway to the detriment of 5-hydroxyindoleacetic acid, producing an accumulation of endogenous melatonin. That suggests, as hypothesized by Martin et al. [234, 239], that the endogenous indoleamines could play a role in the regulation of aqueous humor dynamics (see Section 4.4.4 below).

4.4.2 β-Adrenergic Stimulators

a. Salbutamol and Isoproterenol

The β_1-selective agonists [73] and the β_2-selective agonists, such as salbutamol [70, 203], decrease intraocular pressure after topical application. A variety of explanations, including the desensitization of β-adrenergic receptor adenylcyclase complex [267], have been offered to explain this paradox: Why do both β-agonists and β-antagonists produce ocular hypotensive effects? Yet, any explanation will invite criticism. The most rational explanation is probably that the β_2-agonists, such as salbutamol, increase the outflow facility by activating the β_2-receptors of the trabecular meshwork, the β_2 being the only β-receptors present in that structure. However, the β_1-agonists also decrease intraocular pressure, perhaps, as observed with certain β_1-antagonists, because these agents are not really selective to the ciliary epithelium, but in fact to β_1 and β_2!

In 1955, Weekers et al. [381] first tested the pressure-lowering effect of isoprenaline (isoproterenol), a β_1- and β_2-agonist. Some years later, Weekers and Collignon-Brach [379] observed that isoprenaline (isoproterenol) in its racemic form decreased human intraocular pressure by more than 6 mmHg after 6 hours, and that an effect was observable for up to 48 hours.

However, many side effects make this agent useless; this has since been confirmed by several other authors [33, 175, 327, 338]. Brubaker and Gaasterland [56] in a fluorophotometry study of aqueous humor flow in humans found no measurable effect of isoproterenol on the flow and concluded that this drug may act on the uveoscleral flow.

4.4.3 Arachidonic Acid Metabolites

The early work of Magendie (1824) and Bernard (1858) [225] established that the rabbit eye responds to trauma and nerve injury in a characteristic fashion. More recent articles by Duke-Elder and Duke-Elder [100], Davson and Quilliam [90], and Davson and Huber [89] defined the observable events in response to trauma: miosis, local ocular vasodilatation, increased capillary permeability with a rise in plasma protein content of the aqueous humor, and increase of intraocular pressure. This led Ambache [8] to search for a chemical mediator of this breakdown of the blood-aqueous barrier in the rabbit eye. He named the substance extracted from iris "irin." In 1964, Änggard and Samuelsson [12] presumed that irin could contain prostaglandins (PG) and isolated prostaglandins F2α from sheep iris. Waitzman and King [374] observed the effect of prostaglandins on intraocular pressure.

Thereafter, the ophthalmological literature became rich in reports on the effects of these substances on ocular parameters [45].

Arachidonic acid has three major pathways of metabolization: the cyclooxygenase-dependent pathway, containing prostaglandins, prostacyclins, and tromboxans; the lipooxygenase-dependent pathway, containing lipoxins, mono-HETE, di-HETE, and leukotrienes mainly; and the cytochrome P450 monooxygenase-dependent pathway, containing 12-(R)-HETE and 12-hydroxyeicosatrienoic acid [251].

One should recall that human anterior uvea is able to synthesize all cyclooxygenase products and all lipooxygenase products from arachidonic acids [202]. In this chapter, only the metabolites of interest in aqueous humor dynamics and especially those with hypotensive properties will be treated[2].

4.4.3.1 Cyclooxygenase-Dependent Pathway

a. Prostaglandins F2α and Analogue

First identified in sheep iris by Änggard and Samuelsson [12], prostaglandin F2α (PGF2α) has been studied in the rabbit [29], cat [206], dog [279], monkey [181], and humans [6, 139, 208].

Mechanism of Action

In order to determine the mechanism of action of a drug capable of decreasing intraocular pressure, aqueous humor inflow and outflow must be investigated.

Concerning inflow, Lee, Podos, and Severin [206] observed no change in inflow measured by fluorophotometry and no significant increase in outflow facility measured by tonography in the rabbit, cat, and monkey. Camras et al. [59, 61] found a reduction in outflow resistance in the anesthetized rabbit and no alteration of the aqueous flow as measured by fluorophotometry in the

2 Not every author makes the distinction between prostanoids and eicosanoids. Some use the term eicosanoids for all prostaglandins, leukotrienes, and related compounds because they are derived from 20-carbon essential fatty acids that contain three, four, or five double bonds: 8, 11, 14-eicosatrienoic acid (dihomo-gamma-linolenic acid), and 5, 8, 11, 14, 17-eicosapentaenoic acid.

Cynomolgus monkey. In humans, Kerstetter et al. [185] also found no clinically significant effect on aqueous humor flow and concluded that the reduction of intraocular pressure must be mediated via the outflow system.

One of the first studies on outflow in humans was conducted by Martin [232], who investigated the effect of indomethacin on diurnal variations of intraocular pressure in normal subjects. The result was an increase of the amplitude of diurnal variation of intraocular pressure, suggesting a decrease in outflow facility attributed to blockage by indomethacin of the prostaglandin synthesis normally present in trabecular meshwork cells.

In animals, the laboratories of Bill [294, 295, 296], Bito [44], Kaufman, and their associates [83, 84, 134] have conducted the main studies. The hypothesis that PGs could decrease intraocular pressure by increasing the uveoscleral outflow was suggested by Bito [44] and confirmed by Nilsson et al. [294, 295, 296]. However, uveoscleral outflow increase is not the only site of PGF2α action on aqueous humor dynamics. Indeed, PGF2α increases aqueous humor formation at its beginning [296] and perhaps the episcleral venous pressure through vasodilatation of scleral and conjunctival vessels as well [353].

Prostanoid-Receptors and Intraocular Pressure Reduction

According to Kennedy et al. [183], every naturally occurring prostaglandin has its own receptor, namely, DP for prostaglandin D, EP for PGE, FP for PGF, IP for PGI, and TP for thromboxane. EP receptors are subdivided into three subtypes, EP1, EP2, and EP3.

Goh et al. [140, 141, 142] and Woodward et al. [391] found that stimulation of DP receptors could decrease intraocular pressure in rabbits. In the same species, Waterbury et al. [377] observed that FP, TP, and EP2 receptors do not participate in intraocular pressure lowering, but that selective stimulation of EP3 receptors gives rise to a potent and long-lasting decrease in intraocular pressure.

While part of the site of action now seems to be established, the mechanism itself remains unclear.

Because pilocarpine, known to block uveoscleral flow by contraction of the ciliary muscle [37], is able to prevent the hypotensive effect of PGF2α [83, 84], the mechanism could be a relaxation of the ciliary muscle. The morphological studies of Lütjen-Drecoll and Tamm [222, 223] support this hypothesis. In these studies, the authors found that the ciliary muscle has a relaxed appearance, and that the spaces between ciliary muscle fiber bundles are enlarged. Moreover, a loss of extracellular material was also present. Therefore, a mechanical and biochemical process could be involved in the uveoscleral outflow increase induced by PGF2α.

Since aceclidine has much less effect on the ciliary musculature than pilocarpine [116, 119, 128], it would probably be useful to compare the effect of both drugs on the those of PGF2α. If aceclidine has about the same antagonist effect as pilocarpine on the intraocular effect of PGF2α, we can expect the main pilocarpine-antagonistic action to be situated at the molecular level; and if aceclidine has little or no action, the mechanism of action could be of mechanical origin. In the mechanical hypothesis, PGF2α could act by relaxing the ciliary muscle. On the other hand, in the biochemical hypothesis, PGF2α could affect both synthesis and degradation of glycosaminoglycans and collagen as observed in the human cervix uteri [172, 298]. Otherwise, morphological and biochemical changes might be combined in the mechanism of action of PGF2α, as suggested by the morphological studies of cynomolgus monkey eyes following pretreatment with this drug [222, 223].

Recently, a new phenyl-substituted analog of a prostaglandin F2α prodrug, latanoprost (13, 14-dihydro-17-phenyl-18, 19, 20-trinor-prostaglandin $F2\alpha_1$-isopropyl ester), previously called PhXA41, was found to be an effective hypotensive agent in normal subjects and glaucoma patients [7, 278, 362]. Compared with baseline measurements, PhXA41 reduces the intraocular pressure by 28% to 36% during 1 day after one drop. This drug produces a mild conjunctival hyperemia in 25% to 31% of the cases and can increases pigmentation of the iris possibly due to stimulation of melanogenesis in iris stromal melanocytes [5].

The uveo-scleral outflow doubles in the treated eye and decreases by two-thirds in the contralateral eye. This important decrease of uveo-scleral outflow in the untreated eye can be interpreted as an attempt by the treated eye to maintain its intraocular pressure, which is transmitted in the contralateral eye through axonal reflex [232].

The ocular hypotensive effect of prostaglandins is explained below in the section on melatonin and its metabolites.

b. Other Prostaglandins

Prostaglandins E3 and D3 significantly lowered intraocular pressure in rabbits. Topical PGE3 caused mild conjunctival hyperemia, but it did not induce conjunctival hyperemia [201].

The side effects of PGs of the E, F, and D types were judged to be too important, the ocular hypotensive effect insufficient, and the duration of action too short, which prompted Bito et al. [42, 43] to investigate prostaglandins of A and B types in comparison with various galenical forms of PGF2α. They found a significant improvement with the new prostaglandin types.

In a recent review of the relevant literature, Camras and Podos [62] concluded that several medical and laser treatments presently used in glaucoma therapy reduced intraocular pressure – at least in part – by stimulating endogenous prostaglandin synthesis. These authors distinguished four lines of evidence leading to their conclusion:

1) prostaglandins are potent ocular hypotensive agents;

2) adrenergic and cholinergic agonists stimulate prostaglandin synthesis by ocular tissues in vitro;

3) epinephrine and argon laser trabeculoplasty (ALT) cause elevation of prostaglandin levels in aqueous humor in vivo;

4) prostaglandin synthesis inhibitors such as indomethacin or flurbiprofen block, or partially inhibit, the reduction of intraocular pressure produced by epinephrine, para-aminoclonidine, forskolin, vanadate, verapamil, arachidonic acid, and ALT in rabbits, cats, monkeys, and/or humans.

They also noted that the treatment of glaucoma patients by epinephrine or ALT could be less effective if these patients were simultaneously to receive aspirin ori indomethacin.

4.4.3.2 Lipoxygenase-Dependent Pathway

Stjernschantz et al. [354] investigated the effects of intracameral injection of several arachidonic acid metabolites of the lipoxygenase-dependent pathway in rabbits, guinea pigs, and cats. The hydroperoxy acids (HPETEs) and the hydroxy acids (HETEs) had no significant effect on intraocular pressure, aqueous humor protein, leukocyte concentration, and pupil diameter. On the other hand, leukotriene B4 (LTB4) produced an accumulation of leucocytes in the aqueous humor, an increase of protein content, and an increase in intraocular pressure in the cat, rabbit, and guinea pig. Leukotriene LTC4 and LTD4 caused an intense, long-lasting, non-muscarinic miosis in cats.

4.4.3.3 Cytochrome P450-Dependent Pathway

The cytochrome P450 system converts arachidonic acid to several oxygenated metabolites: monohydroxyeicosatetraenoic acids (HETEs) and epoxyeicosatrienoic (EETs), which can undergo hydrolysis by epoxide hydroxylase to form diol derivatives and omega and omega-1 hydroxylation products. The formation of these metabolites is strictly dependent on nicotinamide-adenine-dinucleotide and on molecular oxygen [251].

In a series of experiments on the corneal epithelium, Schwartzman et al. [332] found that 12(R)-hydroxyeicosa-tetraenoic acid (12-R-HETE), a cytochrom P450-dependent arachidonic acid metabolite produced by the cornea, is a potent inhibitor of Na^+K^+-ATPase. While investigating the effect of 12-R-HETE on intraocular pressure in normotensive rabbits, the same authors measured a significant intraocular pressure-lowering effect, which was maintained for 9 days after single topical application. No sign of inflammation was observed. Because the effect observed with 12-R-HETE was comparable to ouabain injected intravitreally, the authors concluded that 12-R-HETE could act through Na^+K^+-ATPase inhibition [333].

4.4.4 Melatonin and its Metabolites

The first description of melatonin and its metabolites (Fig. 17) in aqueous humor was made in 1988 by Martin et al. [234, 235, 236], who found a mean concentration of 0.47 ng/ml in human aqueous humor. This low concentration of melatonin contrasted with the high concentrations of serotonin (52.5 ng/ml) and 6-hydroxymelatonin (13.9 ng/ml) (Tab. 7).

Because serotonin and certain of its metabolites were seen to be simultaneously present, though at very different levels, in aqueous humor sampled during the day, those authors suggested that there is a circadian rhythm of indoleamines in human aqueous humor. Therefore, we can expect that the amount of melatonin is high and the amount of serotonin low during the night. If serotonin is involved in aqueous humor secretion and aqueous humor flow being about twice as high during the day, melatonin and its metabolites could increase the resistance of outflow during the night, which would explain why intraocular pressure unlike the flow does not drop by 50%.

In 1990 and 1992, Martin et al. [239, 242] published a study showing that the ciliary body was the third organ, after the pineal gland and the retina, found to synthesize indoleamines in humans.

As far back as 1921, Köllner [192] proposed that the alternation of day and night could play a role in the diurnal variations of intraocular pressure. For a while thereafter, this idea was abandoned until Chiou and McLaughlin [67] correlated the diurnal changes in intraocular pressure and the fluctuation of melatonin level in the rabbit eye and suggested that some melatonergic mechanism was involved in the circadian rhythm of intraocular pressure.

Subsequently, serotonin and melatonin were used topically and in intracameral injections. However, while Chiou et al. [66] found no changes in intraocular pressure after intracameral injection of serotonin in rabbit, Krootila et al. [196] observed a rise in intraocular pressure and a breakdown of the blood-aqueous barrier in the same animal. On the other hand, intracameral melatonin produced a significant rise in intraocular pressure, while topical application of melatonin did not affect intraocular pressure, presumably because it did not pass through the cornea sufficiently [66]. Aimoto et al. [3] investigated N-ace-

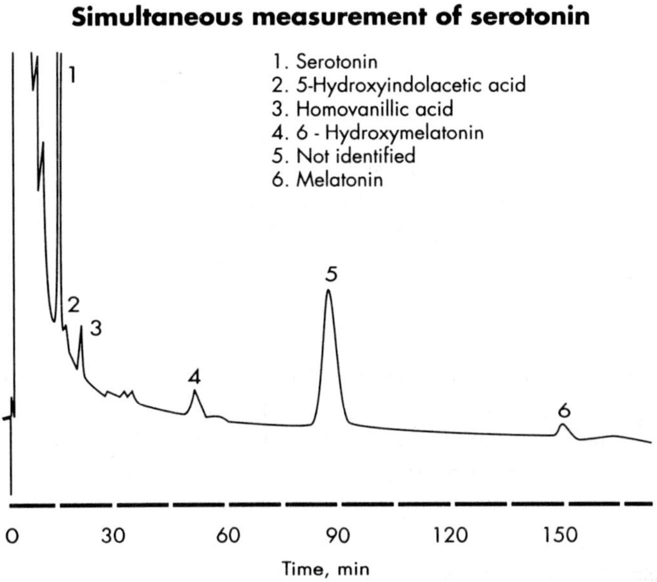

Figure 17. Simultaneous measurement of serotonin, 6-hydroxymelatonin, and melatonin in human aqueous humor using HPLC with electrochemical detection.

Table 7. Serotonin, melatonin, and 6-hydroxymelatonin simultaneously measured in human aqueous humor.

Patient No	Sex	Age (yrs)	Time (o'clock)	Concentration in ng/ml 5-HT	Melatonin	6-OH-Mel
1	M	59	08:10	55.62	2.3	15.18
2	F	23	08:15	35.06	N.D.	8.86
3	M	67	08:35	37.60	N.D.	1.27
4	M	80	08:40	54.82	0.18	19.54
5	F	60	09:00	62.18	0.10	24.00
6	F	71	09:20	63.10	N.M.	12.65
7	M	86	09:30	29.34	N.D.	21.65
8	F	73	10:50	48.45	0.045	2.34
9	F	74	11:15	43.40	0.03*	27.23
10	M	78	12:00	52.20	N.D.	12.06
11	M	82	12:20	46.17	N.M.	8.47
12	F	62	14:15	56.70	0.16	13.62
Mean		67.9		48.72	0.47	13.89
SD		15.9		±10.28	±0.82	±7.76

N.D. = not detected; N.M. = not measured; * less than 3 times the background noise; 5-HT = 5-hydroxytryptamine = serotonin; 6-OH-Mel = 6-hydroxymelatonin.

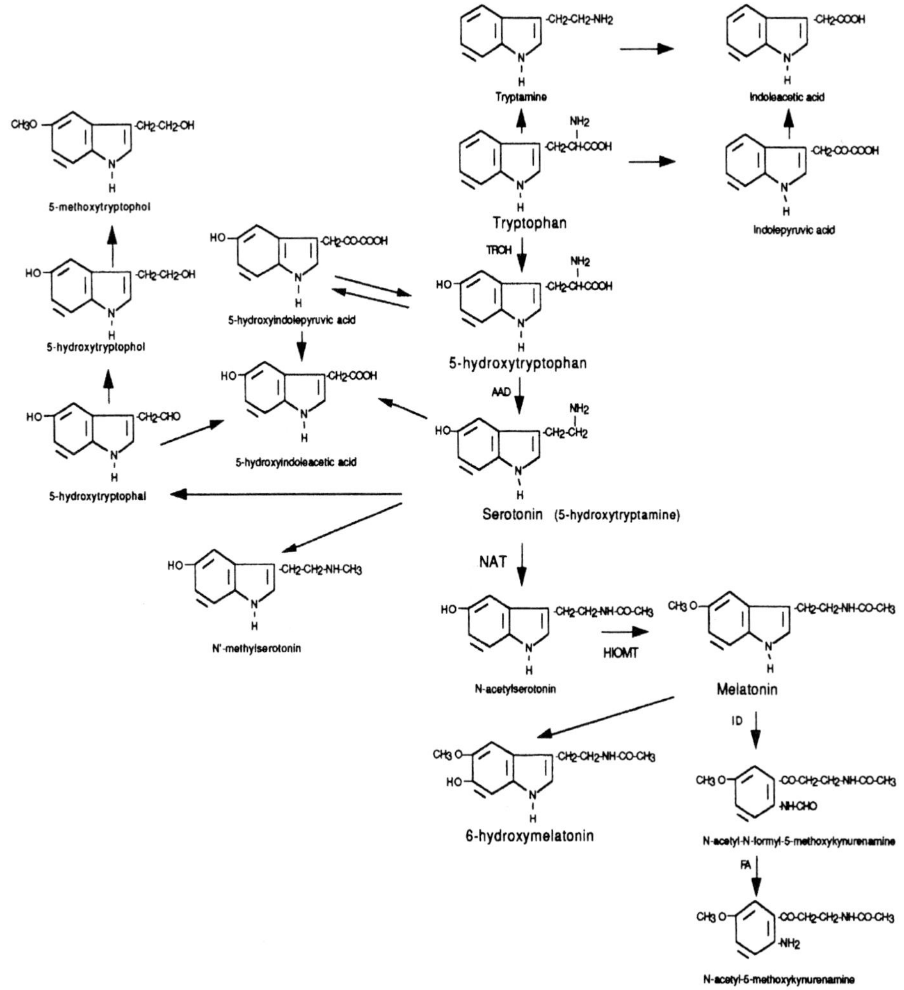

Figure 18. Tryptophan metabolism pathway. Tryptophan, 5-hydroxytryptophan, serotonin, melatonin, 6-hydroxymelatonin, N-acetyl-N-formyl-5-methoxykynurenamine, N-acetyl-5-methoxy-kynurenamine, and the enzymes N-acetyltransferase (NAT) and hydroxyindole-O-methyl-transferase (HIOMT) are the compounds investigated by the author in human aqueous humor and iris-ciliary body. TROH = tryptophan hydroxylase; AAD = L-aromatic acid decarboxylase; ID = indole 2,3-dioxygenase; FA = foraminidase.

tyltransferase activity in normal, preglaucomatous, and glaucomatous chicken eyes, and measured an increase of this enzymatic activity corresponding well to the decrease in aqueous outflow facility.

Rohde et al. [323] observed in the rabbit that pinealectomy had no effect on melatonin concentrations in the ciliary body, and that the diurnal rhythm continued to be observed in this tissue, with values higher at night. In the same study, those authors noticed that intracameral infusion of melatonin into cat eyes produced a decrease of aqueous humor formation and a greater decrease in outflow facility, leading to a significant increase in intraocular pressure. In an attempt to understand whether ocular melatonin was regulated by the adrenergic system as in the pineal gland, the same authors [322] examined the effects of L-timolol, norepinephrine, forskolin, domperidone, and pilocarpine on melatonin concentrations in rabbit and chicken iris-ciliary body. They found no changes in melatonin content in these tissues and suggested that norepinephrine could not be the only transmitter that regulates N-acetyltransferase activity. In humans, however, Brennan et al. [53], in a double-blind study, found a 54% decrease in serotonin concentration in aqueous humor 1 week after beginning timolol 0.5% instillation twice a day in one eye.

Although orally administered melatonin has been reported to lower intraocular pressure in humans [212, 330], it seems more likely that melatonin and certain of its metabolites in fact decrease the outflow facility during the night to maintain ocular pressure, the mean flow suppression being 45% during sleep at night [319]. Because melatonin and especially two of its metabolites (N-acetyl-N-formyl-5-methoxy kynurenamine and N-acetyl-5-methoxykynurenamine; cf. Fig. 18) have some structural and functional similarities with indomethacin, a potent prostaglandin inhibitor; and because N-acetyl-5-methoxy kynurenamine was found by Kelly et al. [182] to be a potent inhibitor of prostaglandin biosynthesis, it is possible that N-acetyl-5-methoxy kynurenamine inhibits endogenous prostaglandin biosynthesis during the night, thus giving rise to a decrease in uveoscleral facility of outflow [233, 243]. Another metabolite of melatonin, 5-methoxytryptamine, is a potent agonist of presynaptic 5-hydroxytryptamine autoreceptors modulating serotonin release [135] and might also be involved in this regulation, albeit only during the day: It was found to be in phase with serotonin and in opposite phase to melatonin (see Section 4.4.1, f. Pargyline, p. 84).

In conclusion, the foregoing permits the suggestion that serotonin (see 4.2.2.1, L-timolol, p. 47) is probably involved in the regulation of the aqueous humor inflow, and that melatonin and some other metabolites are involved in the regulation of aqueous humor outflow [233].

References

1. Aberg G, Welin I. Interaction of β-receptor blocking agents with the nerve blocking effects of procaine in vitro. Life Sci 1967; 6:975–981.
2. Adamek, R. Neue Aspekte zur Glaukomtherapie mit Adrenalin und Adrenalinderivaten. Klin Mbl Augenheilk 1980; 176: 978–981.
3. Aimoto T, Rhode BH, Chiou GC, Lauber JK. N-acetyl-transferase activity and melatonin level in the eyes of glaucomatous chickens. J Ocul Pharmacol 1985; 1:149–160.
4. Airaksinen PJ, Alanko HI. Vascular effects of timolol and pilocarpine in the iris. A simultaneous bilateral fluorescein angiographic study. Acta Ophthalmol 1983; 61:195–205.
5. Alm A, Stjernschantz J. The Scandinavian Latanoprost Study Group. Effects on intraocular pressure and side effects of 0.005% latanoprost applied once daily, evening or morning. A comparison with timolol. Ophthalmology 1995; 102:1743–1752.
6. Alm A, Villumsen J. Intraocular pressure and ocular side effects after prostaglandin F2α eye drops. A single-dose response study in humans. Proc Int Soc Eye Res 1986; 4:3.
7. Alm A, Villumsen J, Törnquist P, Mandahl A, Airaksinen J, Tuulonen A, Marsk A, Resul B, Stjernschantz J. Intraocular pressure-reducing effect of PhXA41 in patients with increased eye pressure. Ophthalmology 1993; 100:1312–1317.
8. Ambache N. Properties of irin, a physiological constituent of the rabbit's iris. J Physiol (London) 1957; 135:114–132.
9. Anderson JA, Davis WL, Wei CP. Site of ocular hydrolysis of a prodrug, dipivefrin, and a comparison of its ocular metabolism with that of parent compound, epinephrine. Invest Ophthalmol Vis Sci 1980; 19:817–823.
10. Anderson L, Wilson WS. Inhibition by indomethacin of the increased facility of outflow induced by adrenaline. Exp Eye Res 1990; 50:119–126.
11. Andréasson S, Moller Jensen K. Effect of pindolol on intraocular pressure in glaucoma: pilot study and a randomised comparison with timolol. Br J Ophthalmol 1983;67:228–230.
12. Änggard E, Samuelsson B. Smooth muscle stimulating lipids in sheep iris. The identification of prostaglandin F2α. Biochem Pharmacol 1964; 13:281–283.
13. Anonymous Adverse systemic effects from ophthalmic drugs. Med Lett Drugs Ther 1981; 24:53–54.
14. Anonymous Phenylephrine eye drops and β-blockers, Med Mett Drugs Ther 1982; 24:70.
15. Badian M, Dabrowski J, Grigoleit HG, Lieb W, Lindner E, Rupp W. Über die Wirkung von Forskolin-Augentropfen auf den Augeninnendruck gesunder männlicher Personen. Klin Mbl Augenheilk 1984; 185:522–526.
16. Baldessarini RJ. Drugs and the treatment of psychiatric disorders. In Gilman AG, Goodman LS, Rall TW, Murad F (eds.) Goodman and Gilman's The Pharmacology Basis of Therapeutics, 7th ed. New York: MacMillan Publ. Co, 1985, p. 416.
17. Ballintine EJ. In Newell FW (ed.). Glaucoma: Transactions of the Fifth Conference. New York, Josiah Macy, Jr Foundation 1960; 248.
18. Bárány EH, A pharmacologist look at medical treatment in glaucoma – In retrospect and in prospect. Ophthalmology 1979; 86:80–94.
19. Barrett AM, Cullum VA. The biological properties of the optical isomers of propanolol and their effects on cardiac arrhythmias. Br J Pharmacol 1968; 34:43–55.
20. Bartels SP, Lee SR, Neufeld AH. The effects of forskolin on cyclic AMP, intraocular pressure and aqueous humor formation in rabbits. Curr Eye Res 1987; 6:307–320.

21. Bartels SP, Roth HO, Jumblatt MM, Neufeld AH. pharmacological effects of topical timolol in the rabbit eye. Invest Ophthalmol Vis Sci 1980; 19:1189–1197.

22. Beatty JF, Krupin T, Nichols PF, Becker B. Elevation of intraocular pressure by calcium channel blockers. Arch Ophthalmol 1984; 102:1072–1076.

23. Becker B. Decrease in intraocular pressure in man by a carbonic anhydrase inhibitor, Diamox. Am J Ophthalmol 1954; 37:13–15.

24. Becker B. Hypothermia and aqueous humor dynamics of the rabbit eye. Trans Am Ophthalmol Soc 1960; 58:337–363.

25. Becker B. Vanadate and aqueous humor dynamics. Proctor Lecture. Invest Ophthalmol Vis Sci 1980; 19:1156–1165.

26. Becker B, Ley AP. Epinephrine and acetazolamide in the therapy of the chronic glaucomas. Am J Ophthalmol 1958; 45:639–643.

27. Berrospi H, Leibowitz HM. Betaxolol. A new β-adrenergic blocking agent for the treatment of glaucoma. Arch Ophthalmol 1982; 100:943–946.

28. Berry DP, Van Buskirk ME, Shields MB. Betaxolol and timolol. A comparison of efficacy and side effects. Arch Ophthalmol 1984; 102:42–45.

29. Bethel RA, Eakins KE. The mechanism of the antagonism of experimentally induced ocular hypertension by polyphloretin phosphate. Exp Eye Res 1972; 13:83–91.

30. Bhat SV, Bajwa BS, Dornauer H, De Souza NJ, Fehlhaber HW. Structures and stereochemistry of new labdane diterpenoids from Coleus forskohlii Briq. Tetrahedron Lett 1977; 19: 1669–1672.

31. Bhattacherjee P, Hammond BR. Effect of indomethacin on the ocular hypotensive action of adrenaline in the rabbit. Exp Eye Res 1977; 24:307–313.

32. Bieck PR, Antonin KH, Balon R, Oxenkrug G. Effect of brofaromine and pargyline on human plasma melatonin concentrations. Prog Neuropsychopharmacol Biol Psychiatry 1988; 12:93–101.

33. Bietti G, Virno M, Pecori-Giraldi J, Pellegrino N, Motolese E. Possibility of isoproterenol therapy with soft contact lenses: Ocular hypotension without systemic effects. Ann Ophthalmol 1976; 8:819–822.

34. Bigger JT, Hoffman BF. Antiarrhythmic drugs. In Gilman AG, Goodman LS, Rall TW, Murad F (eds.) Goodman and Gilman's The Pharmacology Basis of Therapeutics, 7th ed. New York: MacMillan, 1985, p. 769.

35. Bill A. The role of ciliary blood flow and ultrafiltration in aqueous humour formation. Exp Eye Res 1973; 16:287–298.

36. Bill A. Effects of acetazolamide and carotid occlusion on the ocular blood flow in unanesthetited rabbits. Invest Ophthalmol 1974; 13:954–958.

37. Bill, A. Effects of atropine and pilocarpine on aqueous humor dynamics in cynomolgus monkeys (Macaca irus). Exp Eye Res 1967; 6:120–125.

38. Bill A, Phillips CI. Uveoscleral drainage of aqueous humour in human eyes. Exp Eye Res 1971; 12:275–281.

39. Bill A, Walinder PE. The effect of pilocarpine on the dynamics of aqueous humor in a primate (Macaca irus). Invest Ophthalmol 1966; 5:170–175.

40. Birdsall NJM, Burgen ASV, Hulme EC. The binding of agonists to brain muscarinic receptors. Mol Pharmacol 1978; 14:723–736.

41. Bischoff P. Erfahrungen mit einem neuen Adrenalinpräparat in der Glaukomtherapie (Dipivalyl-Epinephrin). Klin Mbl Augenheilk 1978; 172: 565–568.

42. Bito LZ, Baroody RA, Miranda OC. Eicosanoids as a new class of ocular hypotensive agents. 1. The apparent therapeutic advantages of derived prostaglandins of the A and B type as compared to primary prostaglandins of E, F, and D type. Exp Eye Res 1987; 44:825–837.

43. Bito LZ, Miranda OC, Tendler MR, Resul B. Eicosanoids as a new class of ocular hypotensive agents. 3. Prostaglandin A2–1-isopropylester is the most potent reported hypotensive agent on feline eyes. Exp Eye Res 1990; 50:419–428.

44. Bito LZ, Prostaglandins, other eicosanoids, and their derivatives as potential antiglaucoma agents. In Drance SM (ed.) Applied Pharmacology in the Medical Treatment of Glaucomas. New York: Grune and Stratton, 1984; 477–505.

45. Bito, LZ, Stjernschantz J. The ocular effects of prostaglandins and other eicosanoids. Progress in Clinical and Biological Research, vol. 312. New York: Alan R. Liss, Inc 1989; 1–514.

46. Bonomi L, Di Comite P. Outflow facility after guanethidine sulfate administration. Arch Ophthalmol 1967; 78:337–340.

47. Bonomi L, Perfetti S, Noya E, Bellucci R, Massa F. Comparison of the effects of nine β-adrenergic blocking agents on intraocular pressure in rabbits. Albrecht v Graefes Arch klin exp Ophthal 1979; 210:1–8.

48. Bonomi L, Ragnetti E. Sull'azione della instillazione diguanetidina sulla ipertensione oculare sperimentale nel coniglio. Boll Oculist 1964; 43:319–325.

49. Bonomi L, Steindler P. Effect of pindolol on intraocular pressure. Br J Ophthalmol 1975; 59:301–303.

50. Bracher D, Dozzi M, Lotmar W. Measurement of vessel width on fundus photographs. Albrecht v. Graefes Arch klin exp Ophthal 1979; 211:35–48.

51. Brazier DJ, Smith SE. Ocular and cardiovascular response to topical carteolol 2% and timolol 0.5% in healthy volunteers. Br. J. Ophthalmol 1988; 72:101–103.

52. Brennan MC, Martin XD. Dopamine and its metabolites in human tears. Invest Ophthalmol Vis Sci 1988; 29 (Suppl):90.

53. Brennan MC, Martin XD, Heinrich T, Lichter PR. Timolol influences serotonin content in human aqueous humor. Invest Ophthalmol Vis Sci 1990; 31 (Suppl):336.

54. Brodwall J, Fischbarg J. The hydraulic conductivity of rabbit ciliary epithelium in vitro. Exp Eye Res 1982; 34:121–129.

55. Bromberg BB, Gregory DS, Sears ML. β-adrenergic receptors in ciliary process of the rabbit. Invest Ophthalmol Vis Sci 1978; 17:1069–1075.

56. Brubaker RF, Gaasterland D. The effect of isoproterenol on aqueous humor formation in humans. Invest Ophthalmol Vis Sci 1984; 25:357–359.

57. Bucheli J, Aeschlimann J, Gloor B. Die Wirkung von Metoprolol-Augentropfen auf den Augeninnendruck. Klin Mbl Augenheilk 1980; 177:146–150.

58. Calissendorf B. Corneal anaesthesia after topical treatment with timolol maleate. Acta ophthalmol 1981; 59:347–349.

59. Camras CB, Bito LZ, Eakins KE. Reduction of intraocular pressure by prostaglandins applied topically to the eyes of conscious rabbits. Invest Ophthalmol Vis Sci 1977; 16:1125–1134.

60. Camras CB, Feldman SG, Podos SM, Christensen RE, Gardner SK, Fazio DT. Inhibition of the epinephrine-induced reduction of intraocular pressure by systemic indomethacin in humans. Am J Ophthalmol 1985; 100:169–175.

61. Camras CB, Podos SM, Rosenthal JS, Lee PY, Severin CH. Multiple dosing of prostaglandin F2α or epinephrine on Cynomolgus monkey eyes. I. Aqueous humor dynamics. Invest Ophthalmol Vis Sci 1987; 28:463–469.

62. Camras CB, Podos SM. The role of endogenous prostaglandins in clinically-used and investigational glaucoma therapy. Prog Clin Biol Res 1989; 312:459–475.

63. Caprioli J, Sears M, Bausher L, Gregory D, Mead A. Forskolin lowers intraocular pressure by reducing aqueous inflow. Invest Ophthalmol Vis Sci 1984; 25:268–277.

64. Chalfie M, Neufeld AH, Zadunaisky JA. Action of epinephrine and other cyclic AMP-mediated agents on the chloride transport of the frog cornea. Invest Ophthalmol 1972; 11:644–650.

65. Chang FW, Burke JA, Potter DE. Mechanism of the ocular hypotensive action of ketanserin. J Ocul Pharmacol 1985; 1:137–147.

66. Chiou GC, Aimoto T, Chiou LY. Melatonergic involvement in diurnal changes in intraocular pressure in rabbit eyes. Ophthalmic Res 1985; 17:373–378.

67. Chiou GCY, McLaughlin MA. Studies on the involvement of melatonergic mechanism in intraocular pressure regulation. Ophthalmic Res 1984; 16:302–306.

68. Chiou GCY, Zhao F, Shen ZF, Li BHP. Effects of d-timolol and l-timolol on ocular blood flow and intraocular pressure. J Ocul Pharmacol 1990; 6:23–30.

69. Coakes RL, Brubaker RF. The mechanism of timolol in lowering intraocular pressure in the normal eye. Arch Ophthalmol 1978; 96:2045–2048.

70. Coakes RL, Siah PB. Effects of adrenergic drugs on aqueous humor dynamics in the normal human eye. I. Salbutamol. Br J Ophthalmol 1984; 68:393–397.

71. Cohen ML, Fuller RW, Kurz KD. LY53857, a selective and potent serotonergic (5-HT_2) receptor antagonist, does not lower blood pressure in the spontaneously hypertensive rat. J Pharmacol Exp Ther 1983; 227:327–332.

72. Cohen ML, Schenk KW, Kurz KD. 5-ht_2-receptor antagonists: α_1- vs. 5-HT_2-receptor blocking properties in blood vessels. J Cardiovasc Pharmacol 1988; 11:25–29.

73. Colasanti BK, Trotter RR. Effects of selective β_1-and β_2-adrenoreceptor agonists and antagonists on intraocular pressure in the cat. Invest Ophthalmol Vis Sci 1981; 20:69–76.

74. Cole DF. Electrochemical changes associated with the formation of the aqueous humor. Br J Ophthalmol 1961; 45:202–217.

75. Cole DF. Secretion of the aqueous humour. Exp Eye Res 1977; 25 (Suppl):161–176.

76. Collignon N, Guillaume S, Collignon-Brach J. Effet de deux collyres béta-bloquants, le timolol 0,5% et le bétaxolol 0,5% sur le calibre des artères et veines rétiniennes. VIIème Symposium International du Comité de Lutte contre le Glaucome, Reims, octobre 1995.

77. Collignon-Brach J. Long-term effect of ophthalmic β-adrenoceptor antagaonists on intraocular pressure and retinal sensitivity in primary open-angle glaucome. Curr Eye Res 1992; 11:1–3.

78. Collignon-Brach J. Long-term effect of topical β-blockers on intra-ocular and retinal sensitivity in chronic open angle glaucoma. Surv Ophthalmol 1993; 38:149–155.

79. Collignon-Brach J, Weekers R. L'aténolol. Ses effets tensionnels dans le glaucome à angle ouvert. J Fr Ophtalmol 1978; 1:205–210.

80. Collignon-Brach J, Weekers R. Metoprolol et timolol. Etude comparative. J Fr Ophtalmol 1981; 4:275–278.

81. Colloton E, Perkins ES. The effect of timolol on the intraocular pulse pressure. Invest Ophtahlmol Vis Sci 1986; 27 (Suppl):102.

82. Conway JL, Lewis RA. Ocular hypotensive action of ketanserin. Invest Ophthalmol Vis Sci 1988; 30 (Suppl):24.

83. Crawford K, Kaufman PL. Pilocarpine antagonizes prostaglandin F2α-induced ocular hypotension in monkeys. Evidence for enhancement of uveoscleral outflow by prostaglandin F2α. Arch Ophthalmol 1987; 105:1112–1116.

84. Crawford K, Kaufman PL, Gabelt BT. Effects of topical PGF2α on aqueous humor dynamics in cynomolgus monkeys. Curr Eye Res 1987; 6:1035–1044.

85. Cruickshank JM. The clinical importance of cardioselectivity and lipophilicity in β-blockers. Am Heart J 1980; 100:160–178.

86. Dailey RA, Brubaker RF, Bourne WM. The effects of timolol maleate and acetazolamide on the rate of aqueous humor formation in normal human subjects. Am J Ophthalmol 1982; 93:232–237.

87. Dausch D, Gorlich W, Honegger H. Clinical suitability of pindolol eye drops for the treatment of chronic open-angle glaucoma. Klin Mbl Augenheilk 1984; 184:539–542.

88. Davenport HW. The inhibition of carbonic anhydrase by thiophene-2-sulfonamide and sulfanilamide. J Biol Chem 1945; 158:567–571.

89. Davson H, Huber A. Experimental hypertensive uveitis in the rabbit. Ophthalmologica 1950; 120:118–124.

90. Davson H, Quilliam JP. The effects of nitrogen mustard on the permeability of the blood-aqueous humour barrier to Evans blue. Br J Ophthalmo 1947; 31:717–721.

91. Delamere NA, Williams RN. The influence of reserpine and propanolol upon the intraocular response to vanadate in the rabbit. Invest Ophthalmol Vis Sci 1985; 26:1442–1445.

92. Delori FC, Fitch KA, Feke GT, Deupree DM, Weiter JJ. Evaluation of micrometric and microdensitometric methods for measuring the width of retinal vessel images on fundus photographs. Graefe's Arch Clin Exp Ophthalmol 1988; 226: 393–399.

93. Demailly Ph, Aubier G, Abadie P. Timolol et pronostic fonctionnel périmètrique du glaucome primitif à angle ouvert. J Fr Ophthalmol 1985; 8:383–388.

94. Denis Ph. Récepteurs bêta-adrénergiques vasculaires rétiniens chez l'homme. Ophtalmologie 1989; 3:62–64.

95. Draeger J, Schneider, B, Winter R. Die lokal-anästhetische Wirkung von Metipranolol im Vergleich zu Timolol. Klin Mbl Augenheilk 1983; 182:210–213.

96. Draeger J. Corneal Sensitivity. Wien, Springer, 1984

97. Drance SM, Fairclough M, Schulzer M. Dose response of human intraocular pressure to aceclidine. Arch Ophthalmol 1972; 88:394–396.

98. Drayer JI, Weber MA, Frankfort PP. Disparate response of blood pressure to adrenergic stimuli during β-blockage. Gen Pharmacol 1985; 16:229–234.

99. Duffin RM, Christensen RE, Bergamini MVW. Suppression of adrenergic adaptation in the eye with a prostaglandin synthesis inhibitor. Invest Ophthalmol Vis Sci 1981; 21:756–759.

100. Duke-Elder PM, Duke-Elder WS. The vascular responses of the eye. Proc R Soc Lond Ser B 1931; 109:19–28.

101. Duke-Elder S. The formation of aqueous humour. In Duke-Elder S (ed.) System of Ophthalmology, vol. 4. The Physiology of the Eye and of Vision. London: Henry Kimpton, 1968, pp. 186–190.

102. Duke-Elder S. The physiology of the intraocular fluids and its clinical significance. Am J Ophthalmol 1949; 32:1638–1644.

103. Duke-Elder S, Dobree JH. Diseases of the retina. In Duke-Elder S (ed.) System of Ophthalmology, vol 10. Diseases of the Retina. St. Louis: The C.V. Mosby Company 1967, pp. 281–302.

104. Duke-Elder WS. The circulation of intra-ocular fluids. Brit J Ophthalmol 1927; 11:388–392.

105. Duke-Elder WS. The nature of the intra-ocular fluids. Brit J Ophthalmol 1927; 11 (Monograph Suppl):1–140.

106. Duke-Elder WS, Davson H. The present position of the problem of the intra-ocular fluid and pressure. Brit J Ophthalmol 1948; 32:555–569.

107. Duke-Elder WS, Davson H. Studies on the intra-ocular fluids. 1. The reducing substances in the aqueous humour and vitreous body. Brit J Ophthalmol 1949; 33:21–38.

108. Duzman E, Chen CC, Anderson J, Blumenthal M, Twizer H. Diacetyl derivate of nadolol. I. Ocular pharmacology and short-term ocular hypertensive effect in glaucomatous eyes. Arch Ophthalmol 1982; 100:1916–1919.

109. Duzman E, Oner M, Scharrer A, Leopold IH. A clinical evaluation of the effects of topically applied levobunolol and timolol on increased intraocular pressure. Am J Ophthalmol 1982; 94:318–327.

110. Duzman E, Rosen N, Lazar M. Diacetyl nadolol: 3-month ocular hypotensive effect in glaucomatous eyes. Br J Ophthalmol 1983; 67:668–673.

111. Elliot MJ, Cullen PM, Phillips CI. Ocular hypotensive effect of atenolol (Tenormin, I.C.I.). A new β-adrenergic blocker. Br J Ophthalmol 1975; 59:296–300.

112. Epstein DL, Grant WM. Carbonic anhydrase inhibitor side effects: serum chemical analysis. Arch Ophthalmol 1977; 95:1378–1382.

113. Erickson-Lamy K, Schroeder A. Dissociation between the effect of aceclidine on outflow facility and accommodation. Exp Eye Res 1990; 50:143–147.

114. Ericson LA. Twenty-four hourly variations in the inflow of the aqueous humour. Acta Ophthalmol 1958; 36:381–385.

115. Étienne R. Le traitement médical et chirurgical des glaucomes. Marseille, Diffusion Générale de Librairie, 1977; 63.

116. Étienne R, Barut Ch, Gonzalès-Bouchon J. Un nouvel hypotenseur oculaire: l'acéclidine. Ann Oculist (Paris) 1967; 200:287–292.

117. Fahrenbach WH, Bacon DR, Van Buskirk EM. Vasoactive drug effects on the uveal vasculature of the rabbit: a corrosion casting study. Invest Ophthalmol Vis Sci 1989; 30 (Suppl):100.

118. Fechner PU. Vermeidung des Akkommodationsspasmus bei der Behandlung jugendlicher Glaukompatienten. Klin Mbl Augenheilk 1971; 158:112–116.

119. Fechner PU, Teichmann KD, Weyrauch W. Accomodative effects of aceclidine in the treatment of glaucoma. Am J Ophthalmol 1975; 79:104–106.

120. Fechtner RD, Robison MY, Gamero GE, Goldsmith LJ, Zimmerman TJ. A comparison of the efficacy of dorzolamide 2% and oral carbonic anhydrase inhibitors in clinical practice. Invest Ophthalmol Vis Sci 1996; 37 (Suppl):201.

121. Ferrari-Dileo G. β_1- and β_2-adrenergic binding sites in bovine retina and retinal blood vessels. Invest Ophthalmol Vis Sci 1988; 29:695–699.

122. File RR, Patton TF. Topically applied pilocarpine. Human pupillary response as a function of drop size. Arch Ophthalmol 1980; 98:112–115.

123. Fischer FH, Schmitz L, Hoff W, Schartl S, Liegl O, Wiederholt M. Sodium and chloride transport in the isolated human cornea. Pflugers Arch 1978; 373:179–188.

124. Fitzgerald LW, Kaplinsky L, Kimelberg HK. Serotonin metabolism by monoamine oxidase in rat primary astrocyte cultures. J Neurochem 1990; 55:2008–2014.

125. Flammer J, Drance SM. Effect of acetazolamide on the differential threshold. Arch Ophthalmol 1983; 101:1378–1380.

126. Flammer J, Robert, Y, Gloor B. Influence of pindolol and timolol treatment on the visual fields of glaucoma patients. J Ocular Pharmacol 1986; 2:305–311.

127. Flower RJ, Moncada S, Vane JR. Analgesic-antipyretics and anti-inflammatory agents; drugs employed in the treatment of gout. In Gilman AG, Goodman LS, Rall TW, Murad F (eds.) Goodman and Gilman's The pharmacological Basis of Therapeutics. New York: MacMillan Publishing Company, 1985, p. 695.

128. François J, Goes F. Ultrasonographic comparative study of the effect of pilocarpine and aceclidine on the eye components. Ophthalmologica, 1974; 168:299–307.

129. François J, Goes F. Ultrasonographic study of the effect of different miotics on the eye components. Ophthalmologica 1977; 175:328–338.

130. Frauenfelder FT, Meyer, SM. Ocular toxicology. In Duane's Clinical Ophthalmology, Tasman, W, Jaeger, EA (eds.) vol 5, chap 37. J.B. Lippincott Company, Philadelphia, 1993; 15.

131. Friedenwald JS. The formation of the intraocular fluid. Am J Ophthalmol 1949; 32:9–27.

132. Friedenwald JS, Buschke W. The effects of excitements of epinephrine and of sympathectomy on the mitotic activity of the corneal epithelium in rats. Am J Physiol 1944; 141:689–694.

133. Fuller RW, Hemrick-Luecke SK, Kindt MV, Heikkila RE. Different effects of monoamine oxidase inhibition on MPTP depletion of heart and brain catecholamines in mice. Life-Sci 1988; 42:263–271.

134. Gabelt BT, Kaufman PL, Goeckner PA. Direct measurement of increased uveoscleral outflow following PGF2α using two methods. Invest Ophthalmol Vis Sci 1988; 29 (Suppl):127.

135. Galzin AM, Eon MT, Esnaud H, Lee CR, Pevet P, Langer SZ. Day-night rhythm of 5-methoxytryptamine biosynthesis in the pineal gland of the golden hamster (Mesocricetus auratus). J Endocrinol 1988; 118:389–397.

136. Ganong WF. Cardiovascular regulatory mechanisms. In Ganong WF (ed.) Review of Medical Physiology. Los Altos: Lange Medical Publications. 1985; p. 487.

137. Ganong WF. The adrenal medulla and adrenal cortex. In Ganong WF (ed.) Review of medical physiology, 12th ed. Los Altos: Lange Medical Publications, 1985, pp. 296–297.

138. Geyer O, Lazar M, Novack, GD, Shen D, Eto CY. Levobunolol compared with timolol: a four-year study. Br J Ophthalmol 1988; 72:892–896.

139. Giuffrè G. The effects of prostaglandin F2α in the human eye. Graefes Arch Clin Exp Ophthalmol 1985; 222:139–141.

140. Goh Y, Araie M, Nakajima M, Azuma I, Hayaishi O. Effect of topical prostaglandin D2 on the aqueous humor dynamics in rabbits. Graefes Arch Clin Exp Ophthalmol 1989; 227:476–481.

141. Goh Y, Nakajima M, Azuma I, Hayaishi O. Prostaglandin D2 reduces intraocular pressure. Br J Ophthalmol 1988; 72: 461–464.

142. Goh Y, Nakajima M, Azuma, I, Hayaishi O. Effects of prostaglandin D2 and its analogues on intraocular pressure in rabbits. Jpn J Ophthalmol 1988; 32:471–480.

143. Goldmann H. L'origine de l'hypertension oculaire dans le glaucome primitif. Ann Oculist 1951; 184:1086–1105.

144. Goyal RK, Rattan S. Neurohumoral, hormonal, and drug receptors for the lower esophageal sphincter. Gastroenterology 1978; 74:598–619.

145. Grant WM, Trotter PR. Diamox (Acetazoleamide) in treatment of glaucoma. Arch Ophthalmol 1954; 51:735–739.

146. Green K, Kim K. Papaverine and verapamil interaction with prostaglandin E and delta-9-tetrahydrocannabinol in the eye. Exp Eye Res 1977; 24:207–212.

147. Grunwald JE. Effect of timolol on the human retinal circulation. Invest Ophthalmol Vis Sci 1986; 27:1713–1719.

148. Gunning FP, Greve EL, Bron, AM, Bosc JM, Royer JG, George JL, Lesure P, Sirbat D. Two topical carbonic anhydrase inhibitors sezolamide and dorzolamide in Gelrite vehicle: a multilpe-dose efficacy study. Graefe's Arch Clin Exp Ophthalmol 1993; 231:384–388.

149. Hammer R, Berrie CP, Birdsall NJM, Burgen AS, Hulme EC. Pirenzepine distinguishes between different subclasses of muscarinic receptors. Nature 1980; 283:90–92.

150. Hardy. Bull Gén Therap Méd Chir Obst Pharma 1875; 89:458. Cited In Duke-Elder S. System of Ophthalmology, vol. 7. London: Henry Kimpton, 1962; 557.

151. Hass I, Drance SM. Comparison between pilocarpine and timolol on diurnal pressures in open-angle glaucoma. Arch Ophthalmol 1980; 98:480–481.

152. Havener WH. Autonomic drugs. In Havener WH (ed.) Ocular Pharmacology, 5th ed. St. Louis: CV Mosby, 1983; 319.

153. Heilmann K. On the reversibility of the visual field defects in glaucomas. Trans Am Acad Ophthalmol Otolaryngol 1974; 78:304–308.

154. Heilmann K. Das Verhalten des intraokularen Druckes während einer Langzeitbehandlung mit der Kombination Guanethidin-Adrenalin. Klin Mbl Augenheilk 1983; 183: 17–21.

155. Hiramatsu K, Nishimura T, Makiura M, Yamashita H, Uyama M. Morphological changes in the ciliary epithelium after instillation of 0.5% timolol (β-adrenergic blocker). Acta Soc Ophthalmol Jpn 1984; 88:306–1310.

156. Hiramatsu K, Yamashita H. Morphological changes in the ciliary epithelium after subconjunctival administration of befunolol (β-adrenergic blocker). Acta Soc Ophthalmol Jpn 1982; 86:1051–1065.

157. Hiramatsu K, Yamashita H, Uyama M. Morphological changes in the ciliary epithelium after instillation of 1% befunolol (β-adrenergic blocker). Acta Soc Ophthalmol Jpn 1984; 88:251–265.

158. Hitchings RA, Glover D. Adrenaline 1% combined with guanethidine 1% versus adrenaline 1%: a randomised prospective double-blind cross-over study. Br J Ophthalmol 1982; 66:247–249.

159. Hodapp E, Kolker AE, Kass MA, Goldberg I, Becker B, Gordon M. The effect of topical clonidine on intraocular pressure. Arch Ophthalmol 1981; 99:1208–1211.

160. Hoffman BF, Bigger JT. Digitalis and allied cardiac glycosides. In Gilman AG, Goodman LS, Rall TW, Murad F (eds.) G Goodman and Gilman's The Pharmacological Basis of Therapeutics, 7th ed. New York: MacMillan Publishing Company, 1985; 717.

161. Hofmann H. Noradrenalin in der Augenheilkunde. Klin Mbl Augenheilk 1954; 124:63–76.

162. Hogan MJ, Alvarado JA, Weddell JE. Histology of the human eye. Philadelphia: W.B. Saunders Company, 1971, pp. 508–519.

163. Hollands RH, Drance SM, House PH, Schulzer M. Control of intraocular pressure after cataract extraction. Can J Ophthalmol 1990; 25:128–132.

164. Horie T, Takahashi O. Comparison of ocular hypotensive effects of topical timolol and carteolol. Jap J Clin Ophthalmol 1982; 36:1065–1070.

165. Hoyng PhFJ, Dake CL. The aqueous humor dynamics and the biphasic response in intraocular pressure induced by guanethidine and adrenaline in the glaucomatous eye. Albrecht v Graefes Arch klin exp Ophthal 1980; 214:263–268.

166. Innemee HC, Hermans AJM, van Zwieten PA. The influence of clonidine on intraocular pressure after topical application to the eyes of anesthetized cats. Albrecht v Graefes Arch klin Exp Ophthal 1979; 212:19–27.

167. Innemee HC, van Ommeren JD, van Zwieten PA. The influence of acute and chronic cervical sympathectomy on the ocular hypotensive effect of clonidine. Albrecht v Graefes Arch klin exp Ophthal 1979; 212:11–18.

168. Innemee HC, van Zwieten PA. The central ocular hypotensive effect of clonidine. Albrecht v Graefes Arch klin exp Ophthal 1979; 210:93–102.

169. Jaillon P, Heckle J, Weissenburger J, Cheymol G. Comparative dromotropic activity of timolol and propanolol in anesthetized dogs. Eur J Pharmacol 1978; 47:129–134.

170. Janssen PAJ. Serotonin receptors blockage to study serotonin-induced pathology. Trends Pharmacol Sci 1983; 5:198–206.

171. Jay WM, Aziz MZ, Green K. Effect of topical epinephrine and timolol on ocular and optic nerve blood flow in phakic and aphakic rabbit eyes. Curr Eye Res 1984; 3:1199–1202.

172. Joh K, Riede UN, Zahradnick HP. The effect of prostaglandins in the lysomal function in the cervix uteri. Arch Gynec 1983; 234:1–16.

173. Jumblatt JE, North GT. Potentiation of sympathetic neurosecretion by forskolin and cyclic AMP in the rabbit iris-ciliary body. Curr Eye Res 1986; 5:495–502.

174. Kaback MB, Podos SM, Harbin TS, Mandell A, Becker B. The effect of dipivalyl epinephrine on the eye. Am J Ophthalmol 1976; 81:768–772.

175. Kass MA, Reid TW, Neufeld AH, Bausher LP, Sears Ml. The effect of D-isoproterenol on intraocular pressure of the rabbit, monkey, and man. Invest Ophthalmol 1976; 15:113–118.

176. Katz IM, Hubbard WA, Getson AJ, Gould AL. Intraocular pressure decrease in normal volunteers following timolol ophthalmic solution. Invest Ophthalmol Vis Sci 1976; 15:489–492.

177. Katz LJ, Cantor LB, Spaeth GL, Steinmann WC, Samuel F. The short-term effect of a topical β-blocker compared with placebo on perimetry testing in normal subjects. Invest Ophthalmol Vis Sci 1990; 31 (Suppl):149.

178. Kaufman PL, Bárány EH. Loss of acute pilocarpine effect on outflow facility following surgical disinsertion and retro-displacement of ciliary muscle from the scleral spur in the cynomolgus monkey. Invest Ophthalmol 1976; 15:793–807.

179. Kaufman PL, Bárány EH. Residual pilocarpine effects on outflow facility after ciliary muscle disinsertion in the cynomolgus monkey. Invest Ophthalmol 1976; 15:558–561.

180. Keates EU, Stone R. The effect of D-timolol on intraocular pressure in patients with ocular hypertension. Am J Ophthalmol 1984; 98:73–78.

181. Kelly RGM, Starr MS. Effects of prostaglandins and a prostaglandin antagonist on intraocular pressure and protein in the monkey eye. Can J Ophthalmol 1971; 6:205–211.

182. Kelly RW, Amato F, Seamark RF. N-acetyl-5-methoxy kynurenamine, a brain metabolite of melatonin, is a potent inhibitor of prostaglandin biosynthesis. Bioch Biophysical Res Com 1984; 121:372–379.

183. Kennedy I, Coleman RA, Humphrey PPA, Levy GP, Lumley P. Studies on the characterisation of prostanoid receptors: a proposed classification. Prostaglandins 1982; 24:667–689.

184. Kerr CR, Hass I, Drance SM, Walters MB, Schulzer M. Cardiovascular effects of epinephrine and dipivalyl epinephrine applied topically to the eye in patients with glaucoma. Br J Ophthalmol 1982; 66:109–114.

185. Kerstetter JR, Brubaker RF, Wilson SE, Kullerstrand LJ. Prostaglandin F2 α_1-isopropylester lowers intraocular pressure without decreasing aqueous humor flow. Am J Ophthalmol 1988; 105:30–34.

186. Kinsey VE. Comparative chemistry of aqueous humor in posterior and anterior chambers of rabbit eyes. Arch Ophthalmol 1953; 50:401–417.

187. Kinsey VE, Reddy DVN. Turnover of carbon dioxyde in the aqueous humor and the effect thereon of acetazolamide. Arch Ophthalmol 1959; 62:78–83.

188. Kitazawa Y. Long-term glaucoma treatment with MK-507, a topical carbonic anhydrase inhibitor. Ophthalmology 1993; 100 (Suppl):81.

189. Kitazawa Y, Azuma I, Takase M, Komemushi S. Ocular hypotensive effects of carteolol hydrochloride in primary open-angle glaucoma and ocular hypertensive patients. – A double-masked cross-over study for the clinical use -. Acta Soc Ophthalmol Jpn 1981; 85:798–804.

190. Klyce SD, Palkama KA, Härkönen M, Marshall WS, Huhtaniitty S, Mann KP, Neufeld AH. Neural serotonin stimulates chloride transport in the rabbit corneal epithelium. Invest Ophthalmol Vis Sci 1982; 95:1221–1226.

191. Kolker AE, Hetherington J. Becker-Shaffer's Diagnosis and Therapy of the Glaucomas, 5th ed. St. Louis: CV Mosby, 1983; 545–547.

192. Köllner H. Über den Einfluss der Pupillenweite auf den Augendruck beim Glaukom simplex. Arch Augenheilk 1921; 88:58–74.

193. Krieglstein GK. Nadolol eye drops in glaucoma and ocular hypertension: a controlled clinical study of dose response and duration of action. Graefe's Arch Clin Exp Ophthalmol 1981; 217:309–314.

194. Krieglstein GK, Mohamed J. The comparative multiple-dose intraocular pressure responses of nadolol and timolol in glaucoma and ocular hypertension. Acta Ophthalmol 1982; 60:284–292.

195. Krill AE, Newell FW. Effects of pilocarpine on ocular tension dynamics. Am J Ophthalmol 1964; 57:34–41.

196. Krootila K, Palkama A, Uusitalo H. Effect of serotonin and its antagonist (ketanserine) on intraocular pressure in the rabbit. J Ocul Pharmacol 1987; 3:279–290.

197. Krootila K, Uusitalo H, Palkama A. Effect of α-adrenergic and serotonergic blockers on the acute irritative response in the rabbit eye. Exp Eye Res 1987; 45:721–729.

198. Krupin T, Becker B, Podos SM. Topical vanadate lowers intraocular pressure in rabbits. Invest Ophthalmol Vis Sci 1980; 19:1360–1363.

199. Krupin T, Sly WS, Whyte MP, Dodgson SJ. Failure of acetazolamide to decrease intraocular pressure in patients with carbonic anhydrase II deficiency. Am J Ophthalmol 1985; 99:396–399.

200. Küchle HJ. Zur lokalen Wirkung von Guanethidin (Ismelin) auf das gesunde und glaukomkranke Auge. Klin Mbl Augenheilk 1961; 139:224–234.

201. Kulkarni PS, Srinivasan BD. Prostaglandins E3 and D3 lower intraocular pressure. Invest Ophthalmol Vis Sci 1985; 26: 1178–1182.

202. Kulkarni PS, Srinivasan BD. Eicosapentaenoic acid metabolism in human and rabbit anterior uvea. Prostaglandins 1986; 31: 1159–1164.

203. Langham ME, Biggs E. β-adrenergic responses in the eyes of rabbits, primates, and man. Exp Eye Res 1974; 19:281–295.

204. Laties A, Jacobowitz D. Histochemical study of the adrenergic and the cholinergic innervation of the anterior segment of the rabbit eye. Invest Ophthalmol Vis Sci 1964; 3:592–600.

205. Lee PY, Podos SM, Mittag T, Severin C. Effect of topically applied forskolin on aqueous humor dynamics in cynomolgus monkey. Invest Ophthalmol Vis Sci 1984;25:1206–1209.

206. Lee PY, Podos SM, Severin C. Effect of prostaglandin F2α on aqueous humor dynamics of rabbit, cat, and monkey. Invest Ophthalmol Vis Sci 1984; 25:1087–1093.

207. Lee PY, Podos SM, Serle JB, Camras CB, Severin CH. Intraocular pressure effects of multiple doses of drugs applied to glaucomatous monkey eyes. Arch Ophthalmol 1987; 105: 249–252.

208. Lee PY, Shao H, Xu L, Qu, CK. The effect of prostaglandin F2α on intraocular pressure in normotensive human subjects. Invest Ophthalmol Vis Sci 1988; 29:1474–1477.

209. Leenen FHH, Redmond DP, McDonald RH Jr. α- and β-adrenergic induced renin release in man. Clin Pharmacol Ther 1975; 18:31–38.

210. Leopold IH. Current aspects of ocular pharmacology. Surv Ophthalmol 1956; 1:2–34.

211. Leopold IH, Duzman E. Observations on the pharmacology of glaucoma. Ann Rev Pharmacol Toxicol 1986; 26:401–426.

212. Lewy AJ, Sack RL, Miller LS, Hoban TM, Singer CM, Samples JR, Krauss GL. The use of plasma melatonin levels and light in the assessment and treatment of chronobiologic sleep and mood disorders. J Neural Transm 1986; 21 (Suppl):311–322.

213. Lieberman TW, Leopold IH. The use of aceclydine in the treatment of glaucoma. Its effect on intraocular pressure and facility of aqueous humor outflow as compared to that of pilocarpine. Am J Ophthalmol 1967; 64:405–415.

214. Linn DK, Zimmerman TJ, Nardin GF, Yung R, Berberich S, Dubiner H, Fuqua M. Effect of intracameral carbachol on intraocular pressure after cataract extraction. Am J Ophthalmol 1989; 107:133–136.

215. Lish AJ, Camras CB, Podos SM. Effect of apraclonidine on intraocular pressure in glaucoma patients receiving maximally tolerated medications. J Glaucoma 1992; 1:19–22.

216. Liu JHK, Chiou GCY, Garg LC. Ocular hypotensive effects of timolol in cat eyes. Arch Ophthalmol 1980; 98:1467–1469.

217. Liu JHK, Bartels SP, Neufeld AH. Effects of L- and D-timolol on cyclic-AMP synthesis and intraocular pressure in water-loaded, albino and pigmented rabbits. Invest Ophthalmol Vis Sci 1983; 24:1276–1282.

218. Liu JHK, Chiou GCY. Continuous, simultaneous and instant display of aqueous humor dynamics with a microspectro-photometer and a sensitive drop counter. Exp Eye Res 1981; 32:583–592.

219. Lotmar W, Freiburghaus A, Bracher D. measurement of vessel tortuosity on fundus photographs. Albrecht v Graefes Arch klin exp Ophthal 1979; 211:49–57.

220. Lotti VL, LeDouarec J-C, Stone CA. Autonomic nervous system: Adrenergic antagonists. In Sears ML (ed.) Pharmacology of the Eye. Berlin: Springer-Verlag, 1984, pp. 249–267.

221. Lütjen-Drecoll E, Kaufman PL. Biomechanics of echothiophate-induced anatomic changes in monkey aqueous outflow system. Graefe's Arch Clin Exp Ophthalmol 1986; 224:564–575.

222. Lütjen-Drecoll E, Tamm E. Morphological study of the anterior segment of cynomolgus monkey eyes following treatment with prostaglandin F2α. Exp Eye Res 1988; 47:761–769.

223. Lütjen-Drecoll E, Tamm E. The effects of ocular hypotensive doses of PGF2α-isopropylester on anterior segment morphology. In Bito LZ, Stjernschantz J (eds.) The Ocular Effects of Prostaglandins and Other Eicosanoids. New York: Alan R. Liss, Inc, 1989; 437–446.

224. MacIntosh FC. Subtypes of muscarinic receptors: a summary with comments. Trends Pharmacol Sci 1984; 5 (Suppl):100–103.

225. Magendie F. J Physiol Exp (Paris) 1824; 4:176, cited by C. Bernard In Leçons sur la physiologie et la pathologie du système nerveux. 4ème et 5ème leçons, Tome 2. Paris: Baillière, 1858, pp. 48–105.

226. Mandell AI, Stentz F, Kitabchi AE. Dipivalyl epinephrine: a new pro-drug in the treatment of glaucoma. Ophthalmology 1978; 85:268–275.

227. Mannschreck M, Parsons TM, Alvarado JA. Allergic conjunctivitis: a major limitation to the chronic use of apraclonidine. Ophthalmology 1993; 100 (Suppl):81.

228. Maren TH. The relation between enzyme inhibition and physiological response in the carbonic anhydrase system. J Pharmacol Exp Therap 1963; 139:140–153.

229. Maren TH. The rates of movement of Na^+, Cl–, and HCO_3 from plasma to posterior chamber: effect of acetazolamide and a relation to the treatment of glaucoma. Invest Ophthalmol 1976; 15:356–364.

230. Martin X. Agonistes cholinergiques locaux et réactions systémiques paradoxales. J Fr Ophtalmol 1987; 10:129–133.

231. Martin X. Mode d'action des bêta-bloqueurs. Ophtalmologie 1990; 4:154–155.

232. Martin X. Neurosensory control of intraocular pressure in the human eye. A fundamental and clinical correlation. Neuro-ophthalmol 1987; 1:11–25.

233. Martin XD. New insights into the autonomous regulation of intraocular pressure. Curr Op Ophthalmol 1994; 5:15–19.

234. Martin XD, Brennan MC, Lichter PR. Indolamines and aqueous humor regulation. Abstract. Proc Intern Soc Eye Res 1988; 5:73.

235. Martin XD, Brennan MC, Lichter PR. Melatonin in human aqueous humor. Abstract. Proc 3rd Euro Glaucoma Soc 1988; 3:34.

236. Martin XD, Brennan MC, Lichter PR. Serotonin in human aqueous humor. Ophthalmology 1988; 95:1221–1226.

237. Martin XD, Brennan MC, Rabineau PA. Mechanism of action of timolol and aqueous humor secretion. Invest Ophthalmol Vis Sci 1990; 31 (Suppl):182.

238. Martin XD, Brennan MC. Serotonin in human tears. Abstract. Invest Ophthalmol Vis Sci 1989; 30 (Suppl):268.

239. Martin XD, Brennan MC. Diurnal regulation of aqueous humor dynamics. Proc Intern Soc Eye Res 1990; 6:8–9.

240. Martin XD, Brennan MC. Serotonin in human tears. Eur J Ophthalmol 1994; 4:159–165

241. Martin XD, Lichter PR. Neuropharmacologic control of intraocular pressure. In Shields MB, Pollack IP, Kolker AE (eds.) Perspectives in Glaucoma, Transactions of

the First Meeting of the American Glaucoma Society. Thorofare, NJ: Slack, 1988, chap. 11, pp. 113–123.

242. Martin XD, Malina HZ, Brennan MC, Hendrickson, PhH, Lichter PR. The ciliary body – The third organ found to synthesize indoleamines in humans. Eur J Ophthalmol 1992; 2:67–72.

243. Martin XD, Malina HZ. Indoleamines and control of aqueous humor dynamics. Exp Eye Res 1992; 55 (Suppl):44.

244. Martin XD, Malina HZ. N-acetyltransferase activity in human iris-ciliary body. Invest Ophthalmol Vis Sci 1991; 32 (Suppl): 887.

245. Martin XD, Rabineau PA. Can visual field fluctuations be induced by nonselective β-blocker? An analysis by Octopus 500. Invest Ophthalmol Vis Sci 1987; 28 (Suppl):268.

246. Martin XD, Rabineau PA. Intraocular pressure effects of timolol after unilateral instillation. Ophthalmology 1988; 95:1620–1623.

247. Martin X, Rabineau PA. Modifications de l'amplitude des variations nycthémérales sous timolol. J Fr Ophtalmol 1988; 11:843–848.

248. Martin XD, PA Rabineau. Vasoconstrictive effect of topical timolol on human retinal arteries. Abstract. Proc Euro Glaucoma Soc 1988; 3:21.

249. Martin XD, Rabineau PA. Vasoconstrictive effect of topical timolol on human retinal arteries. Graefe's Arch Clin Exp Ophthalmol 1989; 227:526–530.

250. Martin XD, Rabineau PA. Letter to the editor. Graefe's Arch Clin Exp Ophthalmol 1991; 229:299.

251. Masferre JL, Laniado-Chartzman M. Novel cytochrome P450-dependent arachidonic acid metabolites and their ocular effects. In Bito LZ, Stjernschantz J (eds.) The Ocular Effects of Prostaglandins and Other Eicosanoids. Progress in Clinical Biological Research, vol. 312. New York: Alan R. Liss, Inc, 1989, pp. 85–93.

252. Matsuda H, Yoshimura N, Matsumara M, Honda Y. The retinal toxicity of befunolol and other adrenergic β-blocking agents: inhibition of phagocytic activity of cultured retinal pigment epithelial cells. Acta Ophthalmol 1983; 61:343–342.

253. Maxwell RA. Guanethidine after twenty years: a pharmacologist's perspective. Br J Clin Pharmacol 1982; 13:35–44.

254. Maxwell RA, Plummer AJ, Schneider F, Povalski H, Daniel AL. Pharmacology of 2-(octohydro-1-azocinyl)-ethyl guanidine sulfate (SU-5864). J Pharmacol Exp Ther 1960;128:22–29.

255. McCannel CA, Heinrich SR, Brubaker RF. Acetazolamide but not timolol lowers aqueous humor flow in sleeping humans. Graefe's Arch Clin Exp Ophthalmol 1992; 230:518–520.

256. McClure D. The effect of a pro-drug of epinephrine (Dipivalyl epinephrine) in glaucoma-General pharmacology, toxycology, and clinical experience. Am Chem Soc Symp Ser 1975; 224–235.

257. McGoon MD, Vliestra RE, Holmes DR, Osborn JE.The clinical use of verapamil. Mayo Clin Proc 1982; 57:495–501.

258. Mehra KS, Roy PN, Singh R. Pargyline drops in glaucoma. Arch Ophthalmol 1974; 92:453–454.

259. Meldrum NU, Roughton FJW. Some properties of carbonic anhydrase, the CO_2 enzyme present in blood. J Physiol (London) (Proc Physiol Soc) 1932; 75:15P–16P.

260. Meldrum NU, Roughton FJW. Carbonic anhydrase. Its preparation and properties. J Physiol (London) 1933; 80:113–142.

261. Menerath JM, Coulangeon LM, Sole M, Sole P. Aqueous humor flow in normal subjects receiving different β-blockers. International Congress on Fluorophotometry, Luso, Portugal, May 12–13, 1988.

262. Merté HJ, Merkle W. Timolol-Augentropfen in der Glaukombehandlung. Ergebnisse einer Langzeitstudie. Klin Mbl Augenheilk 1980; 170:562–571.

263. Miichi H, Nagataki S. Effects of pilocarpine, salbutamol, and timolol on aqueous humor formation in cynomolgus monkeys. Invest Ophthalmol Vis Sci 1983; 24:1269–1275.

264. Millodot M, Vogel R. The effect of timolol eye drops on corneal sensitivity in pigmented rabbits. Res Clin Forums 1981; 3:79–83.

265. Mishima S. The effects of denervation and the stimulation of the sympathetic and the trigeminal nerve on the mitotic rate of the corneal epithelium in the rabbit. Jpn J Ophthalmol 1957; 1: 65–73.

266. Mithoefer, JC, Mayer PW, Stocks JF. Effect of carbonic anhydrase inhibition on the cerebral circulation of the anesthetised dog. Abstract. Fed Proc 1957; 16:88.

267. Mittag T, Tormay A. Desensitization of the β-adrenergic receptor adenylcyclase complex in rabbit iris-ciliary body induced by topical epinephrine. Exp Eye Res 1981; 33:497–503.

268. Mittag TW, Serle JB, Podos, SM, Cohen L, Liebowitz F. Vanadate effects on ocular pressure, (Na^+, K^+) ATPase and adenylate cyclase in rabbit eyes. Invest Ophthalmol Vis Sci 1984; 25:1335–1338.

269. Mittag TW, Tormay A. Adrenergic receptor subtypes in rabbit iris-ciliary body membranes: classification by radioligand studies. Exp Eye Res 1985; 40:239–249.

270. Monica ML, Hesse RJ, Messerli FH. The effect of calcium channel blocking agent on intraocular pressure. Am J Ophthalmol 1983; 96:814.

271. Morales-Aiguilera A, Williams EMV. The effects on cardiac muscle of β-receptor antagonists in relation to their activity as local anaesthetics. Br J Pharmacol 1965; 24:332–339.

272. Mostaghim R, Maddox YT, Ramwell PW. Endothelial potentiation of relaxation response to β adrenoceptor blocking agents. J Pharmacol Exp Ther 1986; 239:797–801.

273. Mottow-Lippa LS, Lippa EA, Naidoff MA, Clementi R, Bjornsson T, Jones K. 0.008% timolol ophthalmic solution. A minimal-effect dose in normal volunteer model. Arch Ophthalmol 1990; 108:61–64.

274. Murray A, Glover D, Hitchings R. Low-dose combined guanethidine 1% and adrenaline 0.5% in the treatment of chronic simple glaucoma: a prospective study. Br J Ophthalmol 1981; 65:533–535.

275. Musini A, Fabbri B, Bergamaschi M, Mandelli V, Shanks RG. Comparison of the effect of propanolol, lignocaine, and other drugs on normal and raised intraocular pressure in man. Am J Ophthalmol 1971; 72:773–781.

276. Myers MG. β-adrenoceptor antagonism and pressor response to phenylephrine. Clin Pharmacol Ther 1984; 36:57–63.

277. Nagasubramanian S, Hitchings RA, Demailly P, Chuniaud M, Pannarale MR, Pecori-Giraldi J, Stodmeister R, Parsons DG. Comparison of apraclonidine and timolol in chronic open-angle glaucoma. Ophthalmology 1993; 100:1318–1323.

278. Nagasubramanian S, Sheth GP, Hitchings RA, Stjernschantz J. Intraocular pressure-reducing effect of PhXA41 in ocular hypertension. Ophthalmology 1993; 100:1305–1311.

279. Nakano J, Chang ACK, Fisher RG. Effects of prostaglandins E1, E2, A1, A2, and F2α on canine carotid arterial blood flow, cerebrospinal fluid pressure, and intraocular pressure. J Neurosurg 1973; 38:32–39.

280. Namba H. Ocular hypotensive effects and complications of topical befunolol in primary open-angle glaucoma and ocular hypertension. Jap J Clin Ophthalmol 1982; 36:775–781.

281. Nathanson JA. Adrenergic regulation of intraocular pressure; identification of β_2-adrenergic-stimulated adenylate cyclase in the ciliary process epithelium. Proc Natl Acad Sci USA 1980; 77:7420–7424.

282. Nathanson JA. Human ciliary process adrenergic receptor: pharmacological characterization. Invest Ophthalmol Vis Sci 1981; 21:798–804.

283. Nathanson JA. Stereospecificity of β adrenergic antagonists: R-enantiomers show increase selectivity for β_2 receptors in ciliary process. J Pharmacol Exp Ther 1988; 245:94–101.

284. Nathanson JA. Personnal communication, May 10, 1990.

285. Needleman P, Corr PB, Johnson EM. Drugs used for the treatment of angina: organic nitrates, calcium channel blockers, and β-adrenergic antagonists. In Gilman AG, Goodman LS, Rall TW, Murad F (eds.) Goodman and Gilman's The Pharmacological Basis of Therapeutics, 7th ed. New York: Macmillan Publishing Company, 1985, p. 616.

286. Neetens A, Rubbens MC, Van Rompaey J, Hendrata Y. Intraocular pressure lowering effect of timolol in the fellow untreated eye. Bull Soc Belge Ophthalmol 1979; 186: 39–46.

287. Negishi C, Kanai A, Nakajima A, Funahashi M, Kitazawa Y. Ocular effects of β-blocking agent carteolol on healthy volunteers and glaucoma patients. Jpn J Ophthalmol 1981; 25:464–476.

288. Nelson WL, Frauenfelder FT, Stills JM, Arrowsmith JB, Kuritsky JN. Adverse respiratory and cardiovascular events attributed to timolol ophthalmic solution, 1978–1985. Am J Ophthalmol 1986; 102:606–611.

289. Neufeld AH. Experimental studies on the mechanism of action of timolol. Surv Ophthalmol 1979; 186:39–46.

290. Neufeld AH. Glaucoma Editorial. Epinephrine and timolol: How do these drugs lower intraocular pressure? Ann Ophthalmol 1981; 13:1109–1111.

291. Neufeld AH, Page ED. In vitro determination of ability of drugs to bind to adrenergic receptors. Invest Ophthalmol Vis Sci 1977; 16:1118–1124.

292. Nielsen CB, Nielsen PJ. Effect of α- and β-receptor active drugs on corneal thickness. Acta Ophthalmol 1985; 63:351–354.

293. Nielsen NV. Timolol. Hypotensive effect, used alone and in combination for treatement of increased intraocular pressure. Acta ophthalmol 1978; 56:504–509.

294. Nilsson SFE, Sperber GO, Bill A. The effect of prostaglandin F2α_1-iospropylester (PGF2α-IE) on uveoscleral outflow. In Bito LZ, Stjernschantz J (eds). The Ocular Effects of Prostaglandins and Other Eicosanoids. New York: Allan R.Liss, Inc, 1989; 429–436.

295. Nilsson SFE, Stjernschantz J, Bill A. PGF2α increases the uveoscleral outflow. Invest Ophthalmol Vis Sci 1987; 28 (Suppl):284.

296. Nilsson, SFE, Samuelsson M, Bill A, Stjernschantz J. Increased uveoscleral outflow as a possible mechanism of ocular hypotension caused by prostaglandin F2α_1-isopropylester in the cynomolgus monkey. Exp Eye Res 1989; 48:707–716.

297. Nishimura T, Yamashita H, Makiura M, Hiramatsu K, Uyama M. Morphological study on an effect of β-blocker in drug induced ocular hypertension. 2. Ocular hypertension after topically applied prostagalndin E2. Acta Soc Ophthalmol Jpn 1983; 87:818–826.

298. Nordström A. Acute effects of prostaglandins on the biosynthesis of connective tissue constituents in the non-pregnant human cervix uteri. Acta Obstet Gynecol Scand 1984; 63:169–173.

299. Ohrstrom A. Adrenergic β-receptor blockers, adrenalin and intraocular pressure. Acta Ophthalmol 1982; 150 (Suppl):1–58.

300. Pakalnis VA, Rustgi AK, Stefansson E, Wolbarsht ML, Landers MB. The effect of timolol on anterior chamber oxygenation. Ann Ophthalmol 1987; 19:298–300.

301. Palkama A, Uusitalo H, Raij K, Uusitalo R. Comparison of the effects of adrenergic agonists and α, β_1-, β_2-antagonists on the intraocular pressure and adenylate cyclase activity in the ciliary processes of the rabbit. Acta Ophthalmol 1985; 63:9–15.

302. Parver LM, Auker CR, Winkler T, Curtis W, Katan H, Ashburn FS, Doyle T. Effects of timolol on optic nerve head and choroidal blood flow in the cat. Invest Ophthalmol Vis Sci 1985; 26 (Suppl):124.

303. Passo MS, Palmer EA, Van Buskirk EM. Plasma timolol in glaucoma patients. Ophthalmology 1984; 91:1361–1363.

304. Paterson G. Effect of intravenous acetazolamide on relative arcuate scotomas and visual field in glaucoma simplex. Proc Roy Soc Med 1970; 63:865–870.

305. Peczon JD, Grant WM. Diuretic drugs in glaucoma. Am J Ophthalmol 1968; 66:680–683.

306. Phillips CI, Bartholomew RS, Kazi G, Schmitt CJ, Vogel R. Penetration of timolol eye drops into human aqueous humour. Br J Ophthalmol 1981; 65:593–595.

307. Pillunat LE, Stodtmeister R, Wilmanns I, Metzner D. Effect of timolol on optic nerve head autoregulation. Ophthalmologica 1986; 193:146–153.

308. Pilz A, Lommatzsch P, Ulrich WD. Experimentelle und klinische Untersuchungen mit Aceclidin (Glaucostat). Ophthalmologica 1974; 168:376–391.

309. Podos SM, Camras CB, Serle JB. Experimental compounds to lower intraocular pressure. Aust N Z J Ophthalmol 1989; 17:129–135.

310. Podos SM, Lee PY, Severin C, Mittag T. The effect of vanadate on aqueous humor dynamics in cynomolgus monkeys. Invest Ophthalmol Vis Sci 1984; 25:359–361.

311. Pollack FM, de Roetth A. Effect of freezing on the ciliary body (Cyclocryotherapy). Invest Ophthalmol 1964; 3:164–170.

312. Pollack IP. Effect of l-norepinephrine and adrenergic potentiators on aqueous humor dynamics on man. Am J Ophthalmol 1973; 76:641–647.

313. Pollack IP, Becker B, Constant MA, Holmberg A. The effect of hypothermia on aqueous humor dynamics. I. Intraocular pressure and outflow facility of the rabbit eye. II. Ultrastructural changes in the rabbit ciliary epithelium. Am J Ophthalmol 1960; 49: 1126–1140.

314. Pollack IP, Rossi H. Norepinephrine in treatment of ocular hypertension and glaucoma. Arch Ophthalmol 1975; 93:173–177.

315. Radius RL, Diamond GR, Pollack IP, Langham ME. Timolol: a new drug for management of chronic simple glaucoma. Arch Ophthalmol 1978; 96:1003–1008.

316. Rahn KH, Hawlina A, Kersting F, Planz G. Studies on the antihypertensive action of the optical isomers of propanolol in man. Naunyn-Schmiedeberg's Arch Pharmacol 1974; 286: 319–323.

317. Reichert RW, Shields MB, Stewart WC. Intraocular pressure response to replacing pilocarpine with carbachol. Am J Ophthalmol 1988; 106:747–748.

318. Reiss GR, Brubaker RF. The mechanism of betaxolol, a new ocular hypotensive agent. Ophthalmology 1983; 90:1369–1372.

319. Reiss GR, Lee DA, Topper JE, Brubaker RF. Aqueous humor flow during sleep. Invest Ophthalmol Vis Sci 1984; 25:776–778.

320. Richard G, Weber J. Der Einfluss der Betablocker Timolol und Pindolol auf die retinale Hämodynamik-eine videoangiographische Studie. Klin Mbl Augenheilk 1987; 190:34–39.

321. Riley MV. Inhibition by ouabain of glycolysis in ciliary body. Nature (London) 1964; 204:380.

322. Rohde BH, Chiou GC. Is ocular melatonin regulated by adrenergic system? Ophthalmic Res 1987; 19:178–186.

323. Rohde BH, McLaughlin MA, Chiou LY. Existence and role of endogenous ocular melatonin. J Ocul Pharmacol 1985; 1:235–243.

324. Romano JH. Double-blind cross-over comparison of aceclidine and pilocarpine in open-angle glaucoma. Br J Ophthalmol 1970; 54:510–521.

325. Romano JH, Nagasubramanian S, Poinoosawmy D. Double-masked cross-over comparison of Ganda 1.02 (guanethidine 1% and adrenaline 0.2% mixture) with gutt. adrenaline 1% (Simplene 1%) and with pilocarpine 1% (Sno-Pilo 1%). Br J Ophthalmol 1981; 65:50–52.

326. Ros FE, Innemee HC, Van Zwieten PA. Ocular penetration of β-adrenergic blocking agents. An experimental study with atenolol, metoprolol, timolol and propanolol. Doc Ophthalmol 1979; 48:291–301.

327. Ross RA, Drance SM. Effects of topically applied isoproterenol on aqueous dynamics in man. Arch Ophthalmol 1970; 83:39–46.

328. Rowland JM, Potter DE. Adrenergic drugs and intraocular pressure: suppression of ocular hypertension induced by water loading. Exp Eye Res 1980; 30:93–104.

329. Sakimoto G, Une H, Ohba N. Effects of topically applied bupranolol on the intraocular pressure. Effects on the untreated eye. Ophthalmologica 1979; 179:214–219.

330. Samples JR, Krause G, Lewy AJ. Effect of melatonin on intraocular pressure. Curr Eye Res 1988; 7:649–653.

331. Schmitt CJ, Lotti VJ, Le Douarec J-C. Penetration of timolol into the rabbit eye. Measurements after ocular instillation and intravenous injection. Arch Ophthalmol 1980; 98:547–551.

332. Schwarzman ML, Balazy M, Masferrer J, Abraham NG, McGiff JC, Murphy RC. 12(R)-hydroxyeicosatetraenoic acid: a cytochrome P450-dependent arachidonate metabolite that inhibits $Na^{+}K^{+}$-ATPase in the cornea. Proc Natl Acad Sci USA 987; 84:8125–8129.

333. Schwarzman ML, Dunn MW, Masferrer JL. 12(R)hydroxyeicosatetraenoic acid, a novel corneal arachidonate metabolite, lowers intraocular pressure. Invest Ophthalmol Vis Sci 1988; 29 (Suppl):85.

334. Scoville B, Müller B, White BG, Krieglstein GK. A double-masked comparison of carteolol and timolol in ocular hypertension. Am J Ophthalmol 1988; 105:150–154.

335. Sears ML. The mechanism of action of adrenergic drugs in glaucoma. Invest Ophthalmol 1966; 5:115–119.

336. Sears ML, Mead A. A major pathway for regulation of intraocular pressure. Int Ophthalmol 1983; 6:201–212.

337. Sears ML, Neufeld AH. Adrenergic modulation of outflow of aqueous humor. Invest Ophthalmol 1975; 14:83–86.

338. Seidehamel RJ, Dungan KW, Hickey TE. Specific hypotensive and antihypertensive ocular effects of D-isoproterenol in rabbits. Am J Ophthalmol 1975; 79:1018–1025.

339. Seto C, Eguchi S, Araie M, Matsumoto S, Takase M. Acute effects of topical forskolin on aqueous humor humor dynamics in man. Jpn J Ophthalmol 1986; 30:238–244.

340. Share NN, Lotti VJ, Gautheron P, Schmitt C, Gross DM, Hall RA, Stone CA. R-enantiomer of timolol: a potential selective ocular antihypertensive agent. Graefe's Arch Clin Exp Ophthalmol 1984; 221:234–238.

341. Shibata T, Mishima H, Kurokawa T. Ocular pigmentation and intraocular reponse to forskolin. Curr Eye Res 1988; 7:667–674.

342. Shin DH. Bilateral effects of monocular timolol treatment. Am J Ophthalmol 1986; 102:275–276.

343. Shinoara Y. Mechanism of chemical control of cerebral vasomotor activity. Neurology 1973; 23:186–195.

344. Simon KA, Bonting SL, Hawkins NM. Studies on sodium-potassium-activated adenosinetriphosphatase. II. Exp Eye Res 1962; 1:253–261.

345. Smith J, Wandel T. Glaucoma Editorial. Rationale for the one-eye therapeutic trial. Ann Ophthalmol 1986; 18:8.

346. Sonntag JR, Brindley GO, Shields MB. Effect of timolol therapy on outflow facility. Invest Ophthalmol Vis Sci 1978; 17: 293–296.

347. Spinelli D, Montanari P, Vigasio F, Cormanni V. Effets du maléate de timolol sur l'oeil controlatéral sans traitement. J Fr Ophtalmol 1982; 5:153–158.

348. Spinelli D, Vigasio F, Montanari P. Short-term and long-term timolol maleate effects on corneal sensitivity. Doc Ophthalmol 1984; 56:385–392.

349. Staatz WD, Edelhauser HF, Lehner R, Van Horn DL. Cytotoxicity of pivalylphenylephrine and pivalyl acid to corneal endothelium. Arch Ophthalmol 1980; 98:1279–1282.

350. Stenkula E, Wettrell K. A dose-response study of oral atenolol administered once daily in patients with raised intra-ocular pressure. Graefe's Arch Clin Exp Ophthalmol 1982; 218:96–98.

351. Sterk CC. Atenolol 4% eye drops in glaucoma simplex. Doc Ophthalmol 1979; 48:309–314.

352. Stewart RH, Kimbrough RL, Martin PA, Ward RL, Smith JP. Norepinephrine dipivalytate dose-response on ocular hypertensive subjects. Ann Ophthalmol 1981; 13:1279–1283.

353. Stjernschantz J, Nilsson SFE, Astin M. Vasodynamic and angiogenic effects of eicosanoids in the eye. In Bito LZ, Stjernschantz J (eds.) The Ocular Effects of Prostaglandins and Other Eicosanoids. Progress in Clinical and Biological Research, vol. 312. New York: Allan R. Liss, Inc, 1989, pp. 155–170.

354. Stjernschantz J, Sherk T, Borgeat, P, Sears M. Intraocular effects of lipoxygenase pathway products in arachidonic acid metabolism. Acta Ophthalmol 1984; 62:104–111.

355. Takahashi N, Karino S. Long-term treatment of various types of glaucoma with selected β-adrenergic blocking agents. Folia Opthalmol Jpn 1986; 37:741–746.

356. Tane S, Komatsu A, Kubota S. Effect of befunolol ophthalmic solution (a new β-blocking agent in Japan), on lowering intraocular pressure. Folia Ophthalmol Jap 1979; 30:1238–1240.

357. Tervo T, Palkama A. Adrenergic innervation of the rat corneal epithelium. Invest Ophthalmol Vis Sci 1976; 15:147–150.

358. The Levobunolol Study Group. Levobunolol: a β-adrenoceptor antagonist effective in the long-term treatment of glaucoma. Ophthalmol 1985; 92:1271–1276.

359. The Levobunolol Study Group. Levobunolol. A four-year study of efficacy and safety in glaucoma treatment. Ophthalmol 1989; 96:642–645.

360. Tocco DJ, Hooke KF, Deluna FA, Duncan AEW. Stereospecific binding of timolol, a β-adrenergic blocking agent. Drug Met Disp 1976; 4:323–329.

361. Topper JE, Brubaker RF. Effects of timolol, epinephrine, and acetazolamide on aqueous flow during the sleep. Invest Ophthalmol Vis Sci 1985; 26:1315–1319.

362. Toris CB, Camras CB, Yablonski ME. Effects of PhXA41, a new prostaglandin F2α analog, on aqueous humor dynamics in human eyes. Ophthalmology 1993; 100:1297–1304.

363. Tormay A, Ortega M, Mittag T. Calcium/Calmodulin-activated adenylate cyclase in rabbit ciliary process membranes. Invest Ophthalmol Vis Sci 1987; 28 (Suppl): 285.

364. Trope GE, Rumley AG. Catecholamine concentrations in tears. Exp Eye Res 1984; 39:247–250.

365. Tsacopoulos M, David NJ. The effect of arterial PCO2 on relative retinal blood flow in monkeys. Invest Ophthalmol 1973; 12:335–347.

366. Urner-Bloch U, Aeschlimann JE, Gloor BP. Treatment of chronic simple glaucoma with an adrenaline/guanethidine combination at three different dosages (comparative double-blind study). Graefe's Arch Clin Exp Ophthalmol 1980; 213: 175–185.

367. Urner-Bloch U, Bucheli J, Elta H, Gloor B, Aeschlimann J. Klinische Prüfung verschiedener am adrenergen System angreifender Glaukom-Medikamente. Klin Mbl Augenheilk 1980; 176:555–557.

368. Urtti A, Salminen L. A comparison between iris-ciliary body concentration and receptor affinity of timolol. Acta Ophthalmol 1985; 63:16–18.

369. Van Buskirk EM. Corneal anesthesia after timolol maleate therapy. Am J Ophthalmol 1979; 88:864–868.

370. Van Buskirk, EM, Bacon DR, Fahrenbach WH. Ciliary vasoconstriction after topical adrenergic drugs. Am J Ophthalmol 1990; 109:511–517.

371. Van Nueten, JM, Janssen PAJ, Van Beek J, Xhonneux R, Verbeuren TJ, Vanhoutte PM. Vascular effects of ketanserine (R 41 468), a novel antagonist of 5-HT_2 serotonergic receptors. J Pharmacol Exp Ther 1981; 218:217–230.

372. Vareilles P, Silvestone D, Plazonnet B, Le Douarec JC, Sears ML, Stone CA. of the effects of timolol and other adrenergic agents on intraocular pressure in the rabbit. Invest Ophthalmol Vis Sci 1977; 16:987–996.

373. Von Oer S. Über die Beziehung des Acetylcholine des Hornhautepithels zur Erregungsübertragung von diesem auf die sensiblen Nervenenden. Pflügers Arch 1961; 273:325–334.

374. Waitzman MB, King CD. Prostaglandin influences on intraocular pressure and pupil size. Am J Ophthalmol 1967; 212:329–334.

375. Wang RF, Camras CB, Podos SM, Lee KW, Bhuyan KC, Bhuyan DK. The role of prostaglandins in the para-amino-clonidine-induced reduction of intraocular pressure. Trans Am Ophthalmol Soc 1989; 87:94–106.

376. Watanabe K, Chiou GCY. Action mechanism of timolol to lower the intraocular pressure in rabbits. Ophthalmic Res 1983; 15:160–167.

377. Waterbury LD, Eglen RM, Faurot GF, Cooper GF. EP3, but not EP2, FP, or TP prostanoid-receptor stimulation may reduce intraocular pressure. Invest Ophthalmol Vis Sci 1990; 31: 2560–2567.

378. Weber. Korresp-Bl Med Wiss 1876; 14:986. Cited In Duke-Elder S. System of Ophthalmology, vol. 7. The Foundations of Ophthalmology. London: Henry Kimpton, 1962, p. 557.

379. Weekers R, Collignon-Brach J. Etude comparative de diverses amines sympathicomimétiques. Acta Ophthalmol 1966; 44: 762–777.

380. Weekers R, Collignon-Brach J. Bêta-stimulants et bêta-bloquants. Leur place dans le traitement médical du glaucome à angle ouvert. J Fr Ophthalmol 1981; 4:149–155.

381. Weekers R, Demarcelle Y, Gustin J. Treatment of ocular hypertension by adrenalin and diverse sympathomimetic amines. Am J Ophthalmol 1955; 40:666–672.

382. Weekers R, Prijot E, Gustin J. Recent advances and future prospects in the medical treatment of ocular hypertension. Br J Ophthalmol 1954; 38:742–746.

383. Weiner IM, Mudge GH. Diuretics and other agents employed in the mobilization of edema fluid. In Gilman AG, Goodman LS, Rall TW, Murad F (eds.) Goodman and Gilman's The Pharmacological Basis of Therapeutics, 7th ed. New York: Macmillan Publishing Company, 1985; 890–892.

384. Weiner N. Drugs that inhibit adrenergic nerves and block adrenergic receptors. In Gilman AG, Goodman LS, Rall TW, Murad F (eds.) Goodman and Gilman's The Pharmacological Basis of Therapeutics, 7th ed. New York: MacMillan Publishing Company, New York, 1985; 192.

385. Weiner N. Norepinephrine, epinephrine, and the sympathomimetic amines. In Gilman AG, Goodman LS, Rall TW, Murad F (eds.) Goodman and Gilman's The Pharmacological Basis of Therapeutics, 7th ed. New York: MacMillan Publishing Company, 1985, pp. 170–171.

386. Wettrell K, Pandolfi M. Effect of topical atenolol on intraocular pressure. Br J Ophthalmol 1977; 61:334–338.

387. Wilffert B, Davidesco D, DeJonge A, Thoolen M, Timmermans P, Van Zwieten P. Role of ganglionic M_1- and M_2-receptors in the neuronal control of the cardiovascular system of the ormotensive rat as determined with pilocarpine. Eur J Pharmacol 1983; 95:109–116.

388. Wilson TM, Strang R, MacKenzie ET. The response of the choroidal and cerebral circulations to changing arterial pCO2 and acetazolamide in the baboon. Invest Ophthalmol Vis Sci 1977; 16:576–580.

389. Winzerman A, Krey H. Thermographische Untersuchungen zum Wirkungsmechanismus von Timolol. Klin Mbl Augenheilk 1981; 178:190–193.

390. Wistrand PJ. Carbonic anhydrase in the anterior uvea of the rabbit. Acta Physiol Scand 1951; 24:144–148.

391. Woodward DF, Hawley SB, Williams LS, Ralston TR, Protzman CE, Spanda CS, Nieves AL. Studies on the ocular pharmacology of prostaglandin D2. Invest Ophthalmol Vis Sci 1990; 31:138–146.

392. Yablonski ME, Novack GD, Burke PJ, Cook DJ, Harmon G. The effect of levobunolol on aqueous humor dynamics. Exp Eye Res 1987; 44:49–54.

393. Yablonski ME, Zimmerman TJ, Waltman SR, Becker B. A fluorophotometric study of the effect of topical timolol on aqueous humor dynamics. Exp Eye Res 1978; 27: 135–142.

394. Yan HY, Chiou GCY. Effects of L-timolol, D-timolol, haloperidol, and domperidone on rabbit retinal blood flow measured with laser Doppler method. Ophthalmic Res 1987; 19:45–48.

395. Yasuhara H, Sakamoto K, Ueda J. Dissociation between local anesthetic and membrane stabilizing action in antiarrhythmic β-adrenergic blockers and local anesthetics. Anesth Analg 1981; 60:897–990.

396. Yoshida A, Feke GT, Ogasawara H, Goger DG, Murray DL, McMeel JW. Effect of timolol on human retinal, choroidal and optic nerve head circulation. Ophthalmic Res 1991; 23:162–170.

397. Yoshimura K. Activation of Na^+ K^+ activity ATPase in rat brain by catecholamine. J Biochem 1973; 74:289–291.

398. Zeller EA, Shoch D, Cooperman SG, Schnipper RI. Enzymology of the refractory media of the eye. IX. On the role of monoamine oxidase in the regulation of aqueous humor dynamics of the rabbit eye. Invest Ophthalmol 1967; 6:618–623.

399. Zeller EA, Shoch D, Czerner TB, Hsu MY, Knepper PA. Enzymology of the refractory media of the eye. X. Effects of topically administered bradykinin, amine releasers, and pargyline on aqueous humor dynamics. Invest Ophthalmol 1971; 10:274–281.

400. Zimmerman TJ, Harbin R, Pett M, Kaufman HE. Timolol and facility of outflow. Invest Ophthalmol Vis Sci 1977; 16:623–624.

401. Zimmerman TJ, Kaufman HE. Timolol: a β-adrenergic blocking agent for the treatment of glaucoma. Arch Ophthalmol 1977; 95:601–604.

402. Zimmerman TJ, Kaufman HE. Timolol: dose response and duration of action. Arch Ophthalmol 1977; 95:605–607.

CHAPTER 5
CONCLUSION

Although the role of intraocular pressure in the genesis of glaucoma has been known since Pierre Demours and his son, Antoine-Pierre Demours [2], published the first precise description in 1818, its study really began at the end of the 19th century with the first measurements of normal intraocular pressure and its variations. Since then, our knowledge has not ceased to be enriched, though not all regulatory mechanisms of intraocular pressure have been clarified. While intraocular pressure is not the only parameter, it is nevertheless the only one to date that we can measurably influence either surgically or pharmacologically. The pharmacological control of intraocular pressure involves, however, a knowledge of deep-seated mechanisms of aqueous humor dynamics regulation. Today, such knowledge can be acquired only by thorough study of the anatomy, physiology, and pharmacology of the implicated structures. This very step is what motivated the author in his own research as well as in writing the present work.

The findings presented here – not only that indoleamines are present in human aqueous humor and that their respective concentrations vary according to a circadian rhythm, but also that the ciliary body like the pineal gland and the retina is a gland able to synthesize indoleamines in humans (Fig. 19), open up a whole new field of investigation in the understanding of aqueous humor dynamics.

The first pharmacological studies performed to support the hypothetical contribution of indoleamines to the regulation of aqueous humor seem to confirm the important role played by these biogenic amines. Indeed, while a β-blocker such as timolol decreases both intraocular pressure and the amplitude of diurnal variations, this same substance also decreases serotonin concentration in human aqueous humor.

Whereas some arguments permit the theory that some metabolites of serotonin, like melatonin and N-acetyl-5-methoxy kynurenamine, are involved in the regulation of the aqueous humor outflow, this point warrants complementary investigation.

If, however, these results are indeed confirmed, indoleamines could be found to regulate both inflow and outflow. Thus, nature would have created

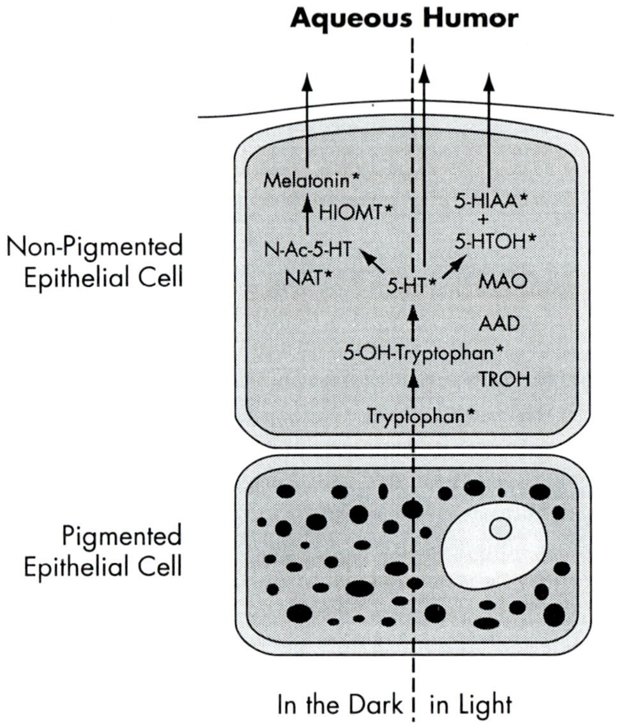

Figure 19. The non-pigmented ciliary epithelial cell and indoleamine synthesis.
In the dark, or during sleep in human, tryptophan is transformed to melatonin and, in the light to other metabolites of serotonin.
Compounds indicated by * were first detected by the author. The nondetection of N-acetylserotonin is explained by the fact that N-acetyltransferase is a limiting enzyme and hydroxyindole-O-methyltransferase and S-adenosyl-L-methionine are present in excess.
TROH = tryptophan hydroxylase; AAD = L-aromatic acid decarboxylase; NAT = N-acetyltransferase; MAO = monoaminooxydase; HIOMT = hydroxyindole-O-methyltransferase.

a regulatory mechanism without redundancy, that is, a mechanism in which each constituent has a single, specific role to play.

These new data advance our knowledge on the physiological mechanism and biochemical cascade involved in aqueous humor dynamics, and they suggest further applications in the control of intraocular pressure. This rational approach merits reflection, since it

1) describes the physiology of the mechanism proposed in the explanation;
2) attempts to influence it with drugs;
3) suggests possible therapeutic applications, rather than carrying out trials with a drug empirically without sufficient knowledge of its possible effects.

Although the results reported here are only fragments of the overall truth, such fragments, according to Claude Bernard [1], are the very building blocks of science.

References

1. Bernard C. Introduction à l'étude de la médecine expérimentale. Réédition de l'édition de 1865. Paris: Garnier-Flammarion, 1966, p. 307.
2. Demours AP. Traité des maladies des yeux, vol. 1. Paris: De l'imprimerie de Firmin Didot, 1818, pp. 468–472.

INDEX